Key Topics in Sexual Health

Steve Baguley
MRCP(UK) BSc DFFP DipGUM
Consultant Genitourinary Physician
Department of Genitourinary Medicine
Woolmanhill Hospital
Aberdeen, UK

Sunil Kumar
MS FRCS(Urol)
Urology Specialist Registrar
Bristol Urological Institute
Southmead Hospital
Bristol, UK

Raj Persad
ChM FRCS(Urol) FEBU
Consultant Urologist and Senior Clinical Lecturer
United Bristol Healthcare Trust
and University of Bristol
Bristol, UK

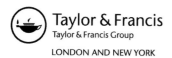

Taylor & Francis
Taylor & Francis Group

LONDON AND NEW YORK

First published in the United Kingdom in 2006 by Taylor & Francis, an imprint of the Taylor & Francis Group, 2 Park Square, Milton Park, Abingdon, Oxon OX14 4RN

Tel.:   +44 (0)20 7017 6000
Fax.:   +44 (0)20 7017 6699
E-mail: info.medicine@tandf.co.uk
Website: www.tandf.co.uk/medicine

Although every effort has been made to ensure that drug doses and other information are presented accurately in this publication, the ultimate responsibility rests with the prescribing physician. Neither the publishers nor the authors can be held responsible for errors or for any consequences arising from the use of information contained herein. For detailed prescribing information or instructions on the use of any product or procedure discussed herein, please consult the prescribing information or instructional material issued by the manufacturer.

A CIP record for this book is available from the British Library.

Library of Congress Cataloging-in-Publication Data

Data available on application

ISBN 1-84184-406-3
ISBN 978-1-84184-406-0

Distributed in North and South America by

Taylor & Francis
2000 NW Corporate Blvd
Boca Raton, FL 33431, USA

Within Continental USA
Tel: 800 272 7737; Fax: 800 374 3401
Outside Continental USA
Tel: 561 994 0555; Fax: 561 361 6018
E-mail: orders@crcpress.com

Distributed in the rest of the world by
Thomson Publishing Services
Cheriton House
North Way
Andover, Hampshire SP10 5BE, UK
Tel.: +44 (0)1264 332424
E-mail: salesorder.tandf@thomsonpublishingservices.co.uk

Composition by Scribe Design, Gillingham
Printed and bound in Great Britain by TJ International, Padstow, Cornwall

Contents

Contributors

Steve Baguley
Consultant Genitourinary Physician
Department of Genitourinary Medicine
Woolmanhill Hospital
Aberdeen, UK

Joan C D Burnett
Associate Specialist in Fertility
Planning and Reproductive Health Care
Square 13 Clinic
Aberdeen, UK

David Cahill
Consultant in Reproductive Medicine
University of Bristol Division of
    Obstetrics and Gynecology
St Michael's Hospital
Bristol, UK

Leslie M Craig
Associate Specialist in Family Planning
    and RHC
Square 13 Clinic
Aberdeen, UK

Tessa Crowley
Associate Specialist in Genitourinary
    Medicine
The Milne Centre for Sexual Health
Bristol, UK

Arnold Fernandes
Consultant in Genitourinary Medicine
Royal United Hospital
Bath, UK

Gillian Flett
Consultant in Sexual and Reproductive
    Health
Foresterhill Hospital
Aberdeen, UK

Kimberley Forbes
Specialist Registrar in Genitourinary
    Medicine
Bart's and The London NHS Trust
London, UK

Venkat Gudi
Consultant Dermatologist
West Suffolk Hospital
Bury St Edmunds
Suffolk

Sunil Kumar
Urology Specialist Registrar
Bristol Urological Institute
Southmead Hospital
Bristol, UK

Andrew Leung
Staff Grade in Genitourinary Medicine
The Milne Centre for Sexual Health
Bristol, UK

Susie Logan
Specialist Registrar in Obstetrics and
    Gynecology
Foresterhill Hospital
Aberdeen, UK

Noel Mack
Associate Specialist in Family Planning
    and RHC
Square 13 Clinic
Aberdeen, UK

Anne MacKenzie
Health Advisor
Genitourinary Medicine
Woolmanhill Hospital
Aberdeen, UK

Gordon McKenna
Consultant in Genitourinary Medicine
Woolmanhill Hospital
Aberdeen, UK

Eileen McKenzie
Health Advisor
Genitourinary Medicine
Woolmanhill Hospital
Aberdeen, UK

Richard Pearcy
Urology Specialist Registrar
Bristol Royal Infirmary
United Bristol Healthcare Trust and
    University of Bristol
Bristol, UK

Raj Persad
Consultant Urologist and Senior
    Clinical Lecturer
United Bristol Healthcare Trust and
    University of Bristol
Bristol, UK

Lindsay Robertson
Consultant Rheumatologist
Derriford Hospital
Plymouth, UK

Paul Sarkar
Specialist Registrar in Genitourinary
    Medicine
Sandyford Initiative
Glasgow, UK

Rachel Thompson
Health Advisor
Genitourinary Medicine
Woolmanhill Hospital
Aberdeen, UK

Sarah Wallage
Consultant in Sexual and Reproductive
    Health
Foresterhill Hospital
Aberdeen, UK

Preface

The World Health Organization's current working definition of sexual health is:

'...a state of physical, emotional, mental and social well-being in relation to sexuality; it is not merely the absence of disease, dysfunction or infirmity. Sexual health requires a positive and respectful approach to sexuality and sexual relationships, as well as the possibility of having pleasurable and safe sexual experiences, free of coercion, discrimination and violence. For sexual health to be attained and maintained, the sexual rights of all persons must be respected, protected and fulfilled.'

Although this oft-quoted definition is rather impenetrable it effectively delivers the message that Sexual Health is about more than just sexually transmitted infections and contraception. Sexual assault, infertility, homophobia, gender dysphoria and sexual harassment are also sexual health issues. As are the sex-lives of such groups as the elderly and those with learning difficulties.

Key Topics in Sexual Health is the product of a multidisciplinary team of urologists, genitourinary physicians and specialists in sexual and reproductive health. It succinctly covers many elements of this diverse field and its structured and readable format makes it a practical guide to the management of many conditions.

The book presents an up-to-date and readable store of practical and relevant information for general practitioners, specialist nurses, practice nurses, trainees in sexual health medicine and non-specialist doctors as well as nursing and medical students.

We hope you enjoy reading it and find it a useful assistant during consultations.

Steve Baguley
Sunil Kumar
Raj Persad
Editors

PART I

THE CONSULTATION AND SEXUAL HISTORY

Sexual history

Paul Sarkar

The sexual history is that part of the consultation that deals with the patient's recent sexual activities. Why should we bother asking someone about their sex life? Well, in this section we will hopefully clarify the usefulness of this line of questioning, even if you do not spend all your time in a sexual health clinic.

Firstly, a sexual history can provide useful information for the differential diagnosis. For example, taking a sexual history from a young woman seen in Accident and Emergency complaining of abdominal pain might allow you to exclude an ectopic pregnancy or make you consider pelvic inflammatory disease. The differential diagnosis of a penile ulcer is quite wide, but if you know that last month he received oral sex from a Gabonese sex worker, then it can remind you to exclude chancroid and syphilis. Secondly, if the person is found to have a sexually transmitted infection (STI), you can immediately tell from the notes how many partners need to be notified. Thirdly, if the history reveals risky sexual practices – consider the returned traveller above – then there can be an opportunity for education and/or hepatitis B vaccination to reduce the chance of further STI acquisition. Finally, the history will indicate which sites need to be sampled – does this gay man have anal sex? If he does, do not assume that he has had *receptive* anal sex – ask him.

A sexual history is more intrusive than other components of the medical history. It is therefore important to put the patient at ease. To maximize the chance of getting an honest account, a patient should be aware that what they say will be treated in confidence, although quite what this means will depend on where you are working. For example, in a genitourinary medicine (GUM) clinic, the details will not end up in a patient's main hospital or primary care notes; a Fraser competent teenager seen in primary care can be pre-emptively reassured that the information will not reach their parents without their consent.

Some people fear that insurance companies will access information. In GUM clinics, such an information release has been prevented by legislation for many years. General practice and hospitals in England, at least, are now covered by similar legislation. The NHS Trusts and Primary Care Trusts (Sexually Transmitted Diseases) Directions of 2000 state that:

> ...information capable of identifying an individual obtained by any of their members or employees with respect to persons examined or treated for any sexually transmitted disease shall not be disclosed except:
>
> a) for the purpose of communicating that information to a medical practitioner, or to a person employed under the direction of a medical practitioner in connection with the treatment of persons suffering from such disease or the prevention of the spread thereof, and
>
> b) for the purpose of such treatment or prevention.

Some people think that you may break confidentiality if they are found to have an infection. In many countries, such as the USA and Australia, STIs are notifiable diseases. This is not the case in the UK. Although their sexual contacts need to be offered testing and treatment, they would not be informed directly without the index case having a chance to do so first (see Partner notification, page 10). Even if informed by the clinician, the partner should not be told who gave their name.

Is the patient comfortable talking to you? If they are looking particularly uneasy during the consultation, ask yourself if they would prefer to talk to someone else, e.g. someone of the same sex. If the consultation is occurring after a sexual assault, such considerations are particularly important.

Is there enough privacy in the consultation area; can people hear through the walls? If you are on a hospital ward, take the person into a side room where you can be alone. Many GUM clinics use a TV or radio to mask the sound of conversation coming through the doors. Is the person accompanied? It is important to give the person a chance to be seen alone. This is particularly important if the other person is a sexual partner or parent.

An appropriate history for someone presenting with genital symptoms or concern about STIs should include:

- their reason for presenting their symptoms
- background information
- their sex life.

Symptoms

If you are working in a sexual health clinic, many people will be asymptomatic and are just there for a sexual health check. However, if they say they have a problem, it is essential to clarify what they mean. Many people resort to vague descriptions when describing their genitals and symptoms. Drawings of the anogenital region can help.

You might think that an 'ulcer' is a break in the skin, but the patient might be using the word to describe their warts. If a man says he has a 'discharge' is it anal, urethral or from under the foreskin?

Once you have both agreed what the symptoms are, ask for some more details – if he has an ulcer, is it painful or painless, single or multiple? What is it associated with: e.g. mouth ulcers, malaise or rash? If the patient has a rash, how did it start, what colour changes occurred, is it itchy? What is it associated with: e.g. mouth lesions, itch everywhere, partner itchy, skin changes on other parts of the body? A picture book may aid diagnosis, particularly if the rash/lump/ulcer has now gone.

Unlike most medical histories it is important to ask direct questions about symptoms since people can be reluctant to report symptoms that they are embarrassed about. Each condition has its characteristic features that can give a clue to the diagnosis from the patient's history – e.g. the discharge of bacterial vaginosis is often smelliest after sex. See the relevant presentation section for further information.

Background information

Ask about past medical history including a history of prior STIs – this would make a diagnosis of an STI on the current visit more likely.

A drug history might help to clarify the cause of symptoms. For example, recent antibiotics might have contributed to the thrush that is causing a woman's itchy discharge. Antibiotics could also suppress the STIs that are about to be tested for, giving false reassurance if the tests are negative. Is the patient taking something that could interact with drugs you might prescribe? Note any drug allergies. Take a note of any contraception used. If a patient is on the combined pill and you prescribe certain antibiotics, she will need to use other methods until 7 days after the course has finished. Could she benefit from a review of her contraception?

If seeing a woman, a gynaecological history is essential – could her pelvic pain be related to the termination she had 2 weeks ago? The last menstrual period is relevant as it might indicate that an episode of unprotected sexual intercourse has resulted in pregnancy. Asking about cervical cytology could throw light on a complaint of intermenstrual bleeding.

When the patient last passed urine is relevant; if it was less than 2 hours ago it will reduce the sensitivity of tests that use a urethral swab and first-void urine specimens.

It can be seen that background information can clarify the existing presentation as well as creating an opportunity for education and prevention of disease and complications of treatment.

Taking a history of sexual activities

It is unusual for someone to decline to answer questions about their recent sex life. However, if you are not working in a sexual health clinic, it can be helpful to introduce this component of the consultation by saying something like, 'I need to ask you some other questions now; they're a bit personal but they will help to clarify what the problem is'. They are unlikely to decline when they see that it is in their own interest to answer the questions.

The questions that need to be asked are:

1. When did you last have sexual contact with anyone? It is better to say 'sexual contact' than 'sex', because some people may not regard activities such as fellatio or masturbation as sex, and therefore may not give a full account.
2. Was that person someone you were going out with or was it just a brief encounter?
3. (If not already clear) What sex was that person?
4. (If they are a regular partner) How long have you been having a sexual relationship with them? The longer they were in a relationship, then the greater the chance of STI transmission.
5. What sort of sex have you had with that person? This indicates which sites need to be sampled. It can also give information about the risk of having acquired an infection; for example, hepatitis C appears to be more common in men who engage in fisting or sadomasochism. Masturbation carries negligible risk of STI acquisition but might have been enough to trigger psychogenic symptoms in someone who regrets an encounter. Ask this question in a way that will be understood by the patient. For example 'receptive anal sex' isn't universally understood and might be met with a puzzled expression. Instead, try asking him if he was 'bottoms' or 'got fucked'.

6. (If appropriate to the encounter) Did you use a condom; was it on all the time?
7. How often do you use condoms with that person? Always, only sometimes?
8. (If heterosexual) Did they use anything else for contraception? If not, this might indicate the need for advice about non-barrier contraception.
9. What was the nationality of the contact? Most STIs are not evenly distributed around the globe, e.g. human immunodeficiency virus (HIV) is 300 times more common in some Southern African countries than in the UK. Likewise antibiotic-resistant strains of gonorrhoea are far more common in South East Asia than in Western Europe.

Then ask, 'When was the last time you had sexual contact with someone else?' and go through the above questions again. It is usual to take this back 3 months or two partners, whichever covers the longer period of time.

With multiple contacts in the previous few months, a sexual history can get quite complex and it helps to document it in a tabular format, as shown in Figure 1.

	When?	Who? (e.g. casual male partner)	Duration (if not just a casual contact)	Activity	Condom last time?	Condoms Always, Usu, Occas, Never	Contra-ception	Nation-ality
Last contact								
Previous								

Figure 1 Tabular format for complex sexual histories

You should now have enough information about the person to know:

• how many people are at risk if you diagnose an infection
• whether they need advice about reducing the risk of future STIs
• which sites to swab.

Following the sexual history, it is usual to ask about risks of acquiring blood-borne viruses. This line of enquiry will also provide information about any historic sexual risks (see Pre-HIV test discussion, page 12).

Adolescents, and child protection

Steve Baguley

The age at which sexual activity is legal varies between countries and a detailed description of what is legal when is beyond the scope of this book. However, regardless of country of residence, people aged 16 and under, who are sexually active are at increased risk of STIs and unplanned pregnancy. Whilst being aware of this and the need to protect them from sexual abuse and exploitation, one must also take into account the natural preference of the young person for a confidential sexual health service.

People don't mature at the same rate and some adolescents could be deemed competent to decide on issues such as the provision of contraception and testing for STIs. In the UK this level of maturity is referred to as Fraser Competence following a ruling on this issue by Lord Fraser in 1985.

In order to decide whether someone has the appropriate maturity the clinician should consider the following issues whilst seeing the patient:

- Do they believe the information you've given them?
- Do you think they able to weigh up the pros and cons of the treatment/management you are suggesting.
- Do you think they have the ability to make a clear choice?
- Have they communicated their decisions to you clearly?

The younger the patient, the less likely it is that they can realistically be regarded as competent. There will also be people aged over 16, perhaps with learning difficulties who will be deemed incompetent to make decisions on sexual health matters.

Even if you decide they are competent, discuss the value of parental support with the young person, but respect their wishes if they do not want to tell their parents. If you decide that they are not competent to decide for themselves you must involve their parent or guardian in any treatment decision.

As well as taking a standard sexual history (see page 3) one must ask about other issues which could increase the chance of the person suffering sexual ill health. In some clinics the receptionist places a card in the notes of any patient aged 16 or under which reminds clinicians of the topics to cover. Use of such a card is encouraged by the UK guideline as a way of ensuring a full and accurate history.

Things to document, issues to cover and questions to ask include:

- Who else is present at the consultation? Is there a risk of coercion from a relative or partner? (Offer to see alone.)
- Age of partner(s). Be aware of possible coercion especially if partner more than 3 years older.
- History of sexual abuse/assault
- Medical and psychiatric history. Depression and low self esteem are associated with unsafe sex.

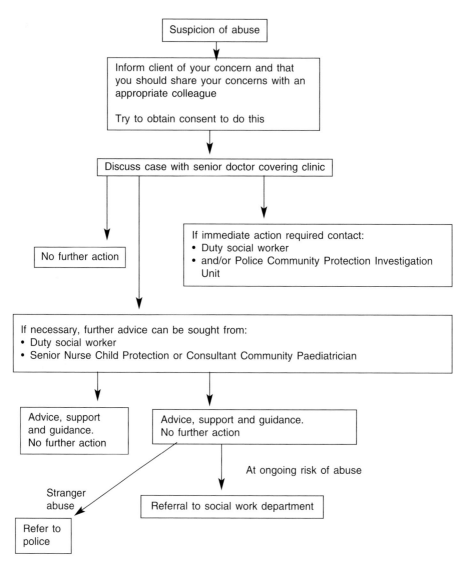

Figure 2 Flow chart for suspected child sexual abuse

- Drug/alcohol use. Most drugs reduce inhibitions. In the UK there appears to be an increase in alcohol consumption by young women.
- Employment/college/school – and whether attending. Sexual ill health is more common in children who are playing truant or who are excluded from school.
- With whom do they live? Both parents? Children's home? There's greater risk of problems in those who are in care.
- Contact with family members if living apart.
- Other agencies, counsellors, support or social workers.

If you are inexperienced in this area discuss any issues raised with a senior colleague. If the child is under 13 they should ideally be seen by two doctors who together decide on their management.

Even if your patient is under the legal age of consent for sexual activity in most instances you are likely to decide that they are competent to accept management without parental involvement and that their sexual relationships are consensual and non-abusive. However, it is important to plan for the day that you realise that your patient is likely to be in an abusive relationship. How you handle this will depend on whether the assailant is resident with the patient and whether the child is at ongoing risk.

Referral pathways will vary between jurisdictions but Figure 2 summarises the approach in the UK and might be of use.

Further reading

Best practice guidance for doctors and other health professionals on the provision of advice and treatment to young people under 16 on contraception, sexual and reproductive health. Department of Health, 29 July 2004

Confidentiality: Protecting and Providing Information. UK General Medical Council. April 2004

Seeking patients' consent: the ethical considerations. UK General Medical Council. November 1998

Thomas A, Forster G, Robinson A and Rogstad K. National Guideline on the Management of Suspected Sexually Infections in Children and Young People. British Association for Sexual Health and HIV. 2003. http://www.bashh.org/guidelines/2002/adolescent_final_0903.pdf [accessed 30/08/2005]

Partner notification (contact tracing)

Eileen McKenzie, Rachel Thompson and Anne MacKenzie

Tracing the sexual contacts of an infected person is an essential element in controlling the spread of STIs through a population. Unlike most conditions, where, once definitively treated the job is done, when you have treated someone for an STI, you are only part way through the management process. Your patient caught the infection from someone and may have passed it on to others. It is your duty to make an attempt to get these people tested and, if necessary, treated. Since many STIs cause symptoms in only a small proportion of infected people, you can not rely on these partners developing symptoms and getting themselves checked up.

Formerly the term 'contact tracing' was used for this process. This term has fallen out of favour because it implies that most sexual contacts have to be tracked down and that the index case (the person with the infection) has no role in the process. For this reason, the term 'partner notification' has become more popular.

The World Health Organisation (1999) describes partner notification as:

...the process of contacting the sexual partners of an individual with a sexually transmitted infection including HIV, and advising them that they have been exposed to infection. By this means, people who are at high risk of STIs/HIV, many of whom are unaware that they have been exposed, are contacted and encouraged to attend for counselling, testing and other prevention and treatment services.

The infections for which partner notification is required include: chlamydia, gonorrhoea, syphilis, trichomoniasis, non-specific urethritis, pelvic inflammatory disease, HIV, hepatitis B, hepatitis C, epididymitis and chancroid.

Partner notification is not required for some STIs, e.g. anogenital warts, molluscum contagiosum and genital herpes. This might seem odd when many of those sexual contacts will be infected with the causative viruses. The problem is that in most cases they will show no signs of the condition and there are no useful diagnostic tests which can detect asymptomatic infection.

Not all of a person's previous sexual contacts need to be notified. The time frame depends on the condition and the mode of presentation. For example, in someone with asymptomatic chlamydia, sexual contacts over the previous 6 months should be notified. In a man with symptomatic urethral gonorrhoea, the time frame is 2 weeks prior to the onset of symptoms. In latent syphilis of unknown duration, partner notification could extend to several years. As you can see, partner notification can vary from a simple matter of a man telling his ex-girlfriend to go and get a check-up to an investigation which attempts to find a dozen people, some of whom may be barely known to the index patient.

When seeing a sexual contact it is important to consider the 'window period' of the infection in question. An HIV test might be negative 2 weeks after a sexual contact with an infected person, but this does not mean that it will still be negative after 3 months.

There are three approaches to partner notification:

1. Partner/client referral. The index patient informs contacts that they need to attend a clinic or their general practitioner (GP) to be screened and possibly undergo treatment.
2. Provider referral. A health care worker informs the patient's contacts that they need to attend a clinic or their GP to be screened and possibly undergo treatment. The contacts are not told the name of the person who gave their details, nor are they told what the infection is.
3. Conditional referral. This is a verbal agreement between the patient and the health care worker that the healthcare worker will inform the contacts if the index has not done so after an agreed number of days.

Resistance to partner notification can be overcome by clarifying the level of confidentiality, e.g. contact data only available to staff involved in care, contacts will not know who gave their details, and contacts will not find out about each other. In order to achieve this, contacts may need to be given appointments at different times.

In the UK, partner notification is usually performed or coordinated by sexual health advisers. These are often people with a background in nursing or a related profession. Health advisers are usually based in GUM clinics. Because of the move toward managing more STIs in primary care and family planning clinics, health advisers are supporting partner notification within these environments.

Another development is centralized partner notification, a system in which details of all relevant STIs diagnosed by a laboratory are forwarded to health advisers. This will include people diagnosed by their GP, those in other community settings and hospital inpatients. Clearly there are issues of consent here – the index patient needs to be aware that their details will be passed on.

As well as detecting previously undiagnosed infection, partner notification is an ideal opportunity to help patients reduce future risk of acquiring an STI. Issues to cover include:

- transmission routes for the various infections
- risk reduction
- factors that may encourage risk taking, e.g. drugs/alcohol, and how to tackle them.

STIs and blood-borne viruses will never be eradicated from a population, but with good partner notification the spread can be limited.

Pre-HIV test discussion

Eileen McKenzie, Rachel Thompson and Anne MacKenzie

In 2004 the English Health Protection Agency estimated that there were about 16 000 people living in the UK who were unaware that they were infected with HIV. Knowledge of the prevalence of undiagnosed infection had previously led to the introduction of an antenatal screening program. In 2001 and 2004 the English/Welsh and Scottish Sexual Health Strategies respectively set targets for an increase in HIV testing by GUM clinics and other settings where STIs are commonly managed. One outcome of these targets has been a debate about how best to increase testing rates. When HIV tests first became available in 1985, there were no effective treatments and to have a test that came back positive was tantamount to a death sentence with an unknown length of time on death row. Some people alleged that they were tested against their will and there was even talk of charging phlebotomists with assault. It was therefore particularly important to gain informed consent for the test.

These days, with reasonably effective antiretrovirals and greatly improved life expectancy, there are very few disadvantages to having a test. Therefore a protracted counselling session before the test is usually unnecessary. However, it is always good practice to inform a patient what investigations you are doing, why you are doing them and what the test involves. This is true whether you are doing thyroid function testing, a chest X-ray or an HIV test. In all these cases, the information should be tailored to the individual with more time spent on those people at risk of getting bad news when they call in to get their results.

Many GUM clinics are choosing to provide information about HIV and its diagnosis in the form of a leaflet. A typical leaflet covers:

- What HIV and acquired immune deficiency syndrome (AIDS) are.
- How you can catch HIV.
- How you can avoid catching HIV.
- The advantages of knowing whether you have HIV, i.e. better prognosis if diagnosed early when antiretrovirals can prevent AIDS and prevention of onward transmission to a fetus or sexual partner.
- Disadvantages of knowing you have HIV. Very few – some difficulty getting business visas for some countries or emigrating to others, distress – could the patient cope at the present time?
- What the test involves.
- The 'window period' (the time taken to develop antibodies following infection).
- How to obtain the result.
- What will happen if the test is negative.
- What will happen if the test is positive.

In GUM clinics, the leaflet is often given to the patient on arrival. In other settings the leaflet can be given to the patient if the clinician feels that a test is indicated.

The consultation

Having read the leaflet, the patient then sees the doctor or nurse. The clinician will establish that the patient has understood the leaflet. If they have not understood it, the information it contains should be reiterated.

During the consultation, the clinician should establish the patient's risk of having HIV. This is done by taking a sexual and risk history. For the sexual history, see page 3. A typical risk assessment might involve asking the following questions:

- Have you ever had sex with someone who has HIV?
- For men: Have you ever had sex with a man?
- For women: Have you ever had sex with a bisexual man?
- Have you ever injected drugs?
- Have you ever had sex with someone who has injected drugs?
- Have you ever had sex with someone from outside the UK? If the answer is yes it is important to find out where the partner was from, since having sex with a Belgian is clearly lower risk than having sex with a Botswanan. UNAIDS collates information on HIV prevalence in each country and produces a useful map.
- Have you ever had a non-professional tattoo or piercing?
- Have you ever had contact with the sex industry? i.e. paid or been paid for sex.

According to the answers to these questions, the clinician assesses the person's risk. In the UK, the main risk factors are sex with someone who has HIV, sex between men and sex with someone from a country where HIV is common. Answering yes to one of these questions would indicate that the person is at increased risk.

If they are perceived to be at increased risk, they should be told so and additional discussion should ensue covering topics such as:

- How will they cope with a positive result?
- Who should they tell about a positive result?
- Testing for other infections (STIs/hepatitides depending on risk group).

If perceived to be at low risk, they should be told so and proceed to testing.

Some clinics ask the patient to sign to say that they consent to have the test, although this is now uncommon.

Even with the increasing prevalence of HIV, most people working in primary care will only very rarely receive a positive result from the lab. This makes it all the more important to have a plan for how you will handle this eventuality. Many 'positive' results are actually false positives, so it is important not to tell the patient the bad news until you have learnt more about the result. The lab will usually ask for a further specimen for confirmation; this is particularly important if not all the components of the test were positive.

Will you refer the patient to your local GUM clinic for the confirmatory test or will you do it yourself? If the confirmatory test is positive, do you have enough information to hand to perform post-test counselling? It is important to have at least thought this through before you offer the patient an HIV test.

With pre-test leaflets and standardized risk assessments, HIV testing will become more routine in primary care. This is a good thing and is essential if the number of undiagnosed cases is to be reduced.

Further reading

Global epidemiology of HIV. Unaids.org.

Rogstad KE, Carter P, Hart GJ et al. UK national guideline on HIV testing. http://www.bashh.org/guidelines/ceguidelines.htm

PART II

PRESENTATIONS

Contraception

At first glance, contraception might seem a simple matter, but many factors can affect the choice for a particular woman. The methods suitable for a healthy teenager are different from those that may be appropriate for an older woman who wishes to space her family. The peri-menopausal period often presents a more complex discussion regarding the best method. The following sections offer a broad-based look at the options available and the factors that may affect the choice of method for each of these groups.

Teenagers

Joan CD Burnett

Teenage girls may seek contraception only when they have already started a sexual relationship. Many will have had unprotected intercourse and may present for the emergency pill or a pregnancy test. This presents an excellent opportunity for the health care professional to discuss contraception and safe sex. They may not wish to embark on hormonal methods on the first visit, but verbal and written information can be given. It is important that the ambience of the clinic is welcoming to young people and that staff are non-judgemental. Opening hours should be as flexible as is practicable and drop-in clinics are particularly useful for this age group. If they feel comfortable with the clinic/surgery setting they are more likely to return for contraceptive advice at a later date.

For those under 16 years of age it is important to consider and assess Fraser competence before prescribing contraception, and this must be documented in the notes. The young person must be assured that the consultation is confidential. However, if there are concerns about an abusive relationship, then the appropriate authorities must be contacted with the teenager's knowledge. Each area should have a child protection officer who can provide assistance in difficult cases. Consent to sex is also a consideration for those with learning difficulties at any age.

It is good practice to ensure that the teenager is happy to have intercourse and does not feel pressured into it by, for example, their boyfriend, peers or the media. Sometimes they need to hear from a health care professional that it is acceptable not to be sexually active if they do not feel ready. By telling them this, they can be empowered to say no and to wait until they are ready.

It is essential to take a medical and family history to establish which methods are suitable. For example, combined contraceptive methods should not be used in those who have focal migraine or a family history of venous thrombosis at a young age. Current medication with liver enzyme inducers (see British National Formulary, BNF), including over-the-counter products like St John's Wort, can render hormonal methods (except Depo-Provera[R]) ineffective and their use needs to be recorded.

The **emergency pill** or Levonelle[R] can be taken up to 72 hours after an episode of unprotected intercourse. Levonelle[R] contains 1500 µg of levonorgestrel and should be taken as soon after the risk episode as possible. The sooner the dose is taken the more effective it is (Table 1). Around 1 in 20 patients may vomit after taking Levonelle[R] and if this occurs within 2 hours of taking the drug they should return for a repeat dose with anti-emetic cover. Liver enzyme-inducing medications such as carbamazepine interact with hormonal methods, and women taking these drugs should take 1500 µg of levonorgestrel as soon as possible, followed 12 hours later by a further 750 µg of the drug.

The patient should be advised to avoid intercourse until after their next period, which may be early or delayed. A pregnancy test is needed 3 weeks after the risk episode unless the patient has had an entirely normal period. Although Levonelle[R] is effective, it is less effective to rely on repeated doses of post-coital contraception than to use an ongoing method.

The copper intra-uterine device (IUD) can also be used as an emergency contraceptive, and this is discussed below (Table 1). However, fitting can be uncomfortable even if the narrow, small Flexi T 300[R] is used. The IUD is 99% effective as emergency contraception and may be preferable to the emergency pill in those who take enzyme inducers or who are at increased risk mid-cycle and present relatively late for the emergency pill. It is the only licensed option for women who present more than 72 hours after the first episode of unprotected sex and may be fitted up to 5 days after predicted ovulation, i.e. up to day 19 of a 28-day cycle. It is an option that should be discussed with any teenager presenting for emergency contraception; however, it is not without risks such as infection and perforation. Therefore, it is usually not the first choice for the majority of teenagers if they are able to take the emergency pill instead. Prophylactic azithromycin 1 g once p.o. should be given when fitting a post-coital IUD when there is a risk of chlamydia infection as well as pregnancy.

Table 1 Risk of pregnancy during a 28-day menstrual cycle and the estimated efficiency of emergency contraception

Risk of pregnancy	
Days 10–17	20–30% risk of pregnancy with unprotected sexual intercourse (UPSI)
Days 1–7 and >17	2–3% risk of pregnancy with UPSI
Estimated efficiency of emergency contraception	
Levonelle within 24 h	95% reduction in expected pregnancies
Levonelle 25–48 h	85% reduction in expected pregnancies
Levonelle 49–72 h	58% reduction in expected pregnancies
IUD up to 5 days after predicted ovulation (i.e. day 19 of 28-day cycle)	>99% reduction in expected pregnancies

Teenagers may be more likely to have multiple partners over relatively short periods of time, so it is important to discuss safer sex and to encourage the use of **condoms**. However, the condom has a high contraceptive failure rate, especially in the inexperienced user, and therefore a more effective method should be used in addition for contraception as fertility is at a peak during the teenage years. Female barrier methods such as the diaphragm require more motivation than most teenagers are willing to put into their contraception and their higher failure rate renders them well down the list of suitable methods for this group.

For the uncomplicated teenage patient, the first choices are the combined pill or patch, injectable progesterone (medroxyprogesterone acetate, Depo-Provera^R) and the etonorgestrel/progesterone implant, Implanon^R. All of these methods prevent ovulation and so offer high levels of contraceptive efficacy when used correctly. Time has to be given to answer the teenager's fears about particular methods and to dispel myths they may have about them.

The **combined oral contraceptive** (COC) consists of oestrogen and a progestogen. The oestrogenic component is usually ethinyloestradiol and the progestogenic component varies. The main serious side effect from the COC is venous thromboembolism. The absolute risk is low: 15–25 per 100 000 women per year compared with 5 per 100 000 women per year for non-users. Individual risk depends on factors such as family history, smoking and body mass index but also with the type of progesterone in the pill. Combined pills containing desogestrel or gestodene have a higher risk than levonorgestrel or norethisterone. The pill with the highest risk, similar to that found in pregnancy (60 per 100 000 women per year), is Dianette^R. This contains the anti-androgen cyproterone, and while often used for women with severe acne or a history of hirsutism, it is not licensed for contraceptive use alone. It may be tried for 6 months before switching to another COC once androgenic symptoms improve. An oestrogen-dominant COC such as Cilest^R may be chosen for women with acne. COC users should be advised to remain active and to avoid dehydration on long-haul flights and to report subsequent symptoms of possible venous thromboembolism urgently.

It is important that time is spent explaining how to take the pill correctly and what to do in the case of missed pills, gastrointestinal upset or concurrent antibiotic use. Minor side effects such as nausea or break through bleeding usually resolve over the first few months and new users need to be aware of this so that they are more likely to persevere. Symptoms that may suggest serious side effects such as pleuritic chest pain or development of focal migraine should be explained and the patient made aware that these require prompt medical attention.

Despite the low failure rate of the method itself (less than 1%), teenage life is often chaotic and it may be difficult for some to comply with pill taking, thus increasing the 'real-life' risk of pregnancy. In this situation it makes sense to use a method that does not rely so heavily on user compliance, e.g. the progestogen injection or implant or the weekly **combined transdermal contraceptive patch**, Evra^R. **Evra^R** offers a welcome alternative for those who want a regular withdrawal bleed but forget pills. See below for more information on this method.

Depo-Provera^R is a high-dose preparation of medroxyprogesterone acetate crystals, which is injected intramuscularly. It gives contraceptive cover for 14 weeks, although injections are usually advised at 12-week intervals. It is not affected by enzyme-inducing drugs. It takes an average of 6 months for fertility to return after stopping Depo-Provera^R. There is a potential risk of osteoporosis in some long-term users. Evidence suggests that bone mass builds up again after use is discontinued, but there are concerns about potential failure to achieve peak bone mass in teenage users. As yet there is no evidence to support this. Depo-Provera^R has a failure rate of less than 1%, slightly superior to that of the COC. Weight gain of around 2–3 kg can occur in about 60% of users due to increased appetite. This can be an issue for many teenagers and requires careful counselling.

The etonorgestrel implant, or **Implanon^R**, is a low-dose progestogenic method. It is a 4 cm by 2 mm flexible rod that is inserted subcutaneously in the upper arm and lasts for 3 years. It releases etonorgestrel at a low rate, which is sufficient to stop ovulation. Unfortunately, it is affected by liver enzyme-inducing drugs and therefore unsuitable as a contraceptive method for those taking these medications. Fertility returns within weeks of removal. It is the most effective method of contraception currently available with a failure rate of less than 0.2%. Slight weight gain occurs in only 10% of users, mostly due to increased appetite. There are few contraindications or serious side effects. No user compliance is necessary once it is fitted, but it does require a minor surgical procedure under local anaesthetic by a suitably trained health care professional for both fitting and removal.

Neither Depo-Provera^R nor Implanon^R are affected by vomiting and diarrhoea or by antibiotic use as they are progesterone-only methods. Unfortunately, the bleeding pattern can be unpredictable initially with both of these methods and the patient needs to be carefully counselled about this before choosing one of these methods. With Depo-Provera, 80–90% of women will have amenorrhoea after the third injection. Around 20% of women continue to have prolonged frequent bleeding after 6 months of implant use. If bleeding is problematical and there are no contraindications, a COC or progesterone-only pill can be used for 2–3 months along with Depo-Provera^R or Implanon^R to regulate the bleeding. Some women choose to continue with the implant long term for contraceptive efficiency even if the bleeding pattern does not settle and use the COC with it for cycle control.

Some teenagers are either unable to tolerate combined methods because of side effects or cannot take it for medical reasons and do not want to use the injection or implant. Other methods are available. The **progesterone-only pill** (POP) can be used, but the 3-hour window for taking most of these pills may be difficult to follow. The POP acts on cervical mucus and endometrium but does not usually prevent ovulation. The real-life pregnancy rate is higher than for other hormonal methods.

If a POP is to be used then it is probably best to use the newer desogestrel preparation Cerazette^R in this age group as it has a 12-hour window and is more likely to stop ovulation. See below for more information about the POP.

The **intrauterine device** (IUD) and the **intrauterine system** (IUS), or Mirena^R, may also be considered. In those who have not had a pregnancy, the uterus may be too small to fit an IUD or IUS. Women without a previous vaginal delivery are also more likely to require local anaesthetic to the neck of the womb to facilitate fitting. Few teenagers will actually choose these methods, but a number will ask about them, especially if they have had problems with hormonal methods and feel that the copper IUD may offer them an effective hormonal-free method. The copper IUD often increases menstrual flow and cramping, whereas the IUS reduces flow once established. (Refer to later sections of this chapter for more information on these methods.)

For some religious groups, hormonal or barrier methods may be unacceptable and natural alternatives such as Billings' method must be discussed and the teenager directed to facilities trained in these methods.

Women in their 20s and 30s

Leslie M Craig

The contraceptive needs of this age group are rarely singled out for discussion but there are probably more sexually active and fertile women requiring an effective method in this age group than in any other.

The number of terminations of pregnancy in this age group is high, showing the importance of contraception for those wishing to avoid or postpone pregnancy.

Women planning pregnancy need advice about reversibility of the different methods. The contraceptive consultation may be a good opportunity to give preconceptual advice about folic acid supplementation and rubella serology for example.

Post-partum women need accurate information about return of fertility. This should be assumed from 21 days post-partum if the baby is bottle fed. If a woman is amenorrhoeic *and* her baby is exclusively **breast fed**, she has 98% natural contraceptive cover for the first 6 months after delivery. She may be concerned about the effects of contraceptive hormones on the baby.

Women in this age group may be involved in shift work, travel across time zones or travel to areas where contraceptive services are limited. Contraceptive methods must be chosen to suit lifestyle factors as well as medical history.

Some issues have been addressed in the section on contraception in teenagers and others will be discussed in the section on women over 40.

Combined contraception

This is the most popular method of contraception for this age group. A 30-year-old woman who has used the pill for over 10 years may be concerned about long-term side effects and the effect of the pill on her fertility. Many unplanned pregnancies occur when women feel they should 'take a break' from the combined pill. Questions about risks and benefits of long-term use and about alternatives need balanced discussion.

See above for information about the risk of venous thromboembolism with COC use.

The relative risk of breast cancer for women using the COC is 1.24. There is also an increased risk of cervical cancer, relative risk 1.3 for 5–9 years' use and 2.5 for 10 or more years' use. These risks return to those of someone who has never used the pill within 10 years of stopping. The overall number of women developing breast or cervical cancer due to combined contraceptive use is small, despite the increased relative risks.

These increases are balanced by a 50% decreased risk of ovarian and endometrial cancer that persists for up to 15 years after stopping the pill and a decreased risk of functional ovarian cysts and benign breast cysts.

A contraceptive consultation is an ideal opportunity to discuss cervical screening and ask about a family history of breast, ovary, bowel or endometrial cancer, which may allow reassurance or prompt referral for genetic advice.

Women can be reassured that there is no evidence that the pill effects long-term fertility. Many women used to regular 'artificial' withdrawal bleeds on combined contraception may notice that their natural menstrual cycles are more irregular when they discontinue.

Combined methods offer several non-contraceptive benefits, including improved acne and premenstrual tension. Withdrawal bleeds are typically lighter, shorter, less painful and more regular than natural periods. Two or three packs can be taken together without a break (bicycling/tricycling) to avoid a withdrawal bleed. This may suit holidays, travel or career commitments.

The transdermal combined contraceptive patch EVRA[R] has a similar efficacy and side effect profile to the combined pill. This relatively new method of contraception involves wearing a patch for a week at a time for 3 weeks then having a patch-free week. A regular withdrawal bleed is likely in the patch-free week. This method may be useful for women who have difficulty remembering to take a pill daily due to child care, travel or shift work commitments and who do not wish to consider injectables or implants or intrauterine contraception.

Combined methods are not recommended for women who are breast feeding, but in women who are bottle feeding it can be started after 6 weeks when the post-partum thromboembolism risk has returned to baseline.

Progestogen-only pill

This has traditionally been used by women for whom the combined pill is contraindicated or causes unacceptable side effects. Traditional progestogen-only pills (POP) contain levonorgestrel, ethynodiol or norethisterone and need to be taken within a 3-hour window, i.e. no more than 27 hours between pills. This may be difficult to adhere to. The new desogestrel POP Cerazette[R] has a 12-hour window and is more likely to prevent ovulation and so is expected to be more effective than a standard POP. The POP has a very low risk of venous or arterial thrombosis and so is suitable for women with a high body mass index (BMI), previous thromboembolism, diabetes, focal migraine or who are smokers over 35 years old. Women may have amenorrhoea, regular cycles or an unpredictable cycle. Side effects may include headaches, breast tenderness or acne, but these are relatively rare due to the low doses involved. The POP can be used during breastfeeding, starting from day 21 post-partum.

Injectable progestogen Depo-Provera[R]

This is a popular method for women in their mid reproductive years who appreciate the high incidence of amenorrhoea after prolonged use. Some women, however, notice weight gain.

There may be an average 6 month delay before fertility returns after the injection runs out. It is therefore important to discuss pregnancy plans before administering Depo-Provera[R], especially for women in their late 30s with naturally declining fertility. Depo-Provera[R] can be used during breast feeding. It does not have an increased thrombosis risk but may cause heavy erratic bleeding if given within 6 weeks of delivery.

Progestogen implant (Implanon[R])

The etonorgestrel rod is an extremely effective contraceptive and fertility returns to baseline status within weeks of implant removal. The time and cost involved with fitting and removal may make it a less appropriate method if pregnancy is planned within a year.

The 3-year duration of action makes the implant a popular method for women going overseas for long periods who may not have easy access to contraceptive supplies.

As with Depo-Provera^R, there is no concern about venous thrombosis with long-haul travel.

Implanon^R can be used during breast feeding and can be fitted from 21 days post-partum.

Intra-uterine device IUD

- Although the IUD can usually be fitted for women who have not had a pregnancy, it becomes a more popular choice after a vaginal delivery as insertion is likely to be easier.
- Fitting is delayed until the first post-partum period or until 6 weeks post-partum in a lactating amenorrhoeic woman to allow uterine involution. It is important to consider the possibility of new pregnancy before inserting a device.
- Modern copper IUDs are 98–99% effective and last for 5–8 years depending on the device chosen.
- Fertility returns to baseline within a cycle after removal.
- The IUD is hormone free, which appeals to many women, and also makes the method suitable for women taking enzyme-inducing drugs.
- Many women notice that their periods are longer, heavier or more crampy with an IUD in situ. Before choosing an IUD, women need to be aware of the 1 in 1000 perforation rate and approximately 15% expulsion rate. These complications are most likely at or soon after insertion.
- The IUD is associated with an increased risk of pelvic infection for 3 weeks after insertion, but subsequent infection is related to STI acquisition rather than the IUD. It is important to discuss a woman's past and ongoing risk of STIs and offer STI screening as appropriate.
- Women with an IUD and their medical attendants should consider pregnancy if pain or abnormal bleeding occurs. If a pregnancy occurs, an urgent ultrasound scan is needed to confirm its site.
- Approximately 20% of pregnancies which occur with an IUD in situ will be extra-uterine. The overall risk of ectopic pregnancy with an IUD remains lower than for a woman using barrier methods as the absolute risk of pregnancy is lower.

Most IUDs are T-shaped frames with copper around the stalk. The Gynefix^R is a frameless device consisting of copper bead-like sleeves on a filament that is anchored in the myometrium at insertion. Initial research studies suggested that this device would cause less dysmenorrhoea and have a lower expulsion rate. However, this has not been borne out in UK practice and there are concerns about higher perforation rates at insertion.

The IUD does not affect breast feeding.

Intra-uterine system (Mirena^R)
This method shares the low failure rate of the copper IUD, but after an initial 3–4 months of erratic bleeding, dramatically reduces menstrual loss. Women may have

light regular bleeds, erratic spotting or amenorrhoea. The incidence of systemic side effects is lower than with other progestogenic methods.

Fertility returns rapidly after removal of the IUS. The Mirena can be used during breast feeding. It can be fitted with the first post-partum period, as for the IUD.

Barrier methods

These methods rely more on the user and her partner than those discussed so far. Quoted real-life failure rates therefore vary from 2–20%.

Male condoms are readily available and raise no concern about reversibility or hormonal side effects. Protection against sexually transmitted infections is relevant to all age groups.

There is no proven increased contraceptive effect from spermicidal condoms, and the nonoxynol-9 may cause vaginal epithelial damage and thus increase transmission of HIV with frequent use. Lubricated but spermicide-free condoms should be recommended. Polyurethane male (Avanti) and female (Femidom) condoms are available if there are concerns about latex sensitivity for either partner.

Many household/medical chemicals such as Vaseline and vegetable oil can damage latex and lead to method failure.

The latex diaphragm or cervical cap is an option for some women. Clinical staff show the woman how to insert the correct size of device to occlude the cervix. The method needs consistent careful use but can be inserted some hours before intercourse. Additional spermicide use is advised in the UK.

It can be fitted 6 weeks post-partum and clearly does not affect breast feeding.

A different size of diaphragm or cap may be needed after a weight change of more than 3 kg, including that during pregnancy.

Emergency contraception

This remains a valuable back-up after unprotected sex or method failure. It can be used during breast feeding; only women who are fully breast feeding and amenorrhoeic in the first 6 months after delivery can assume natural contraceptive protection.

Advance prescription of emergency contraception may be considered for women relying on barrier methods and travelling to areas with limited access to post-coital contraception. See above for more information about the effectiveness of emergency contraception.

Sterilization/vasectomy

Male or female sterilization can be offered to men or women who are sure that their family is complete. Although reversal may be technically possible, both methods should be regarded as irreversible. Counselling must include discussion about the possibility of relationship breakdown or bereavement, in which case a further pregnancy may be desperately wanted. Men or women under 30 years old are usually advised to use an effective but reversible method as the incidence of regret following sterilization is higher in this age range. Many couples wrongly assume that sterilization is 100% effective or is reversible and may not have accurate information about the full range of contraceptive options.

Vasectomy has a 1 in 2000 failure rate once azoospermia is confirmed by semen analysis, usually 3 or 4 months after the procedure. There are no effects on erectile function, cardiovascular disease or prostate or testicular cancer. The operation is usually performed using local anaesthetic.

Female sterilization in the UK is generally performed by tubal occlusion using Filshie clips. Laparoscopy is necessary, with its associated anaesthetic and operative risks. There is a 1 in 200 lifetime failure rate and a subsequent pregnancy may be ectopic. New hysteroscopic methods of tubal occlusion are in limited use; data is still being collected to assess long-term failure rates and side effects.

Female sterilization has no direct effect on the menstrual cycle, but a woman who stops hormonal contraception after sterilization may find that her natural cycles are heavier and less regular.

Contraception in the over 40s

Noel Mack

What is on offer for the more mature woman requiring contraception? She is becoming less fertile but still requires safe, effective, acceptable contraception. We need to remember that both maternal morbidity and mortality and the risk of fetal chromosomal abnormality and miscarriage increase with maternal age.

Menstrual problems become more common in this age group both from dysfunctional bleeding and gynaecological pathology such as fibroids or peri-menopausal anovulatory cycles.

Baseline risks of venous and arterial thrombosis naturally increase with age, as does the incidence of breast cancer.

Women over 40 can continue to use the full range of contraceptive methods in various forms but, as always, need individual discussion about the risks and benefits of each.

Women who have ended a long-term relationship with a partner who has had a vasectomy may be unaware of new contraceptive methods available.

Women using hormonal contraception will not be able to rely on their menstrual cycle to confirm menopause. Two episodes of elevated blood levels of follicle stimulating hormone (FSH) 3 months apart can help support a diagnosis of menopause in women using progestogenic methods. The assay cannot be interpreted for women on combined contraception.

There remains a chance of late ovulation and conception after regular ovulation ceases regardless of FSH levels. Contraception is therefore recommended for 2 years after the menopause in women under 50 and 1 year in women over 50. Women on the POP may prefer to simply continue this extremely low risk method until the age of 55, when infertility can be expected.

Combined contraception

The combined pill (COC) remains a highly effective option for non-smoking, normotensive women up to the age of 50. These women do not have an increased risk of myocardial infarction (MI) or haemorrhagic stroke although they have an increased risk of ischaemic stroke compared to non-users (relative risk 1.5). Smoking or hypertension, however, dramatically increases the risks in non-users and users alike. Thus, smokers over 35 should discontinue combined contraception, and regular blood pressure monitoring should continue for the older woman who continues using COC.

Venous thromboembolism becomes more frequent with age regardless of other risk factors.

The risk of breast cancer is slightly increased (relative risk of 1.24) for current users. As women approach 50, the background incidence of breast cancer is also rising so the absolute numbers affected increase. The risk needs to be addressed in a balanced way, looking at benefits as well as risks from the COC. Breast awareness needs to be emphasized.

The lowest dose should be used to give cycle control. Non-contraceptive benefits of combined contraception may affect choice. These include lighter periods, less dysmenorrhoea, possible improvements in premenstrual syndrome and peri-menopausal symptoms, reduced risk of ovarian and endometrial cancer, possible suppression of endometriosis, and proven maintenance of bone density. The ability to take two packs together (bicycle packs) to postpone a withdrawal bleed is valued by women with travel or work commitments that would make a withdrawal bleed inconvenient.

Progestogen-only methods
There are four progestogen-only methods available in the UK. The progestogen-only pill (**POP**), depot injection (**Depo-Provera^R**), sub-dermal implant (**Implanon^R**), and the intra-uterine system (**Mirena^R**).

These are all safe, effective methods of contraception in this older age group, with no evidence of increased cancer or heart disease risks. They can be used in women with a history of venous thromboembolism (VTE). There is still debate about **Depo-Provera^R** causing low bone density that recovers within 5 years of stopping the method. Alternatives should be discussed with women over 45 or who have other risk factors for low bone density. These include premature menopause, smokers, family history, steroid use, and low body weight (BMI<20). This concern does not apply to the other progestogen-only methods.

The biggest drawback of these methods is the acceptability of what for some can be a chaotic bleeding pattern. Some may become amenorrhoeic. Careful counselling can be very helpful in helping women accept their bleeding pattern. See above for more information on these methods. New irregular bleeding may be caused by gynae-cological pathology and warrants examination and investigation.

The **POP** is a very good choice for the older woman whose reduced fertility gives a failure rate of <1%. It can be difficult to be sure when a woman has gone through the menopause while using POP, so rather than stopping to see, using condoms and having a small but real risk of pregnancy, it is suggested that the POP should be continued until age 55, when 98% of women will be infertile.

The bleeding pattern can be unpredictable, ranging from amenorrhoea to frequent light bleeding. Differentiating between irregular bleeding caused by POP and that caused by underlying disease can be a challenge.

Implanon can also be used in this age group as a safe and effective long-term contraceptive. It may be difficult to tell when a woman goes through the menopause using this method, so remember that fertility returns immediately Implanon is removed. Side effects of bloating, mood changes, headaches or worsening of pre-menstrual/menstrual symptoms may occur around the menopause in some women. These can also occur as a result of using Implanon.

Mirena^R

The progestogen-coated intrauterine system has been discussed in the previous section. In this age group it can be a useful treatment for dysfunctional uterine bleeding. Peri-menopausal women with intolerable vasomotor symptoms may try hormone replacement therapy. This can cause irregular bleeding as there is still some natural ovarian function. The Mirena^R can also be used as the progestogenic part of hormone replacement therapy to prevent endometrial hyperstimulation while oestrogen is administered by the oral or transdermal route. The Mirena^R needs to be changed every 5 years when used in hormone replacement therapy or for contraception in the under 45s. There is some evidence that it will provide effective contraception for 7 years for women who have it fitted over the age of 45. The licence may change in the next few years to reflect this. An amenorrhoeic woman over the age of 52 who is due a contraceptive Mirena^R change may discuss using barrier methods and watching her menstrual cycle to see if she is menopausal, rather than having a new device fitted.

The **Intra-uterine device (IUD)** has been discussed in the previous section. The IUD is hormone free, and as there are no hormonal effects, the end of menstruation is easy to assess. An IUD fitted after the age of 40 will provide effective contraception until the menopause and does not need to be replaced. It will need to remain in place until 1 year after the last menstrual period if the woman is over 50, and for 2 years if the last menstrual period is when the woman is under 50. The IUD often increases menstrual flow and dysmenorrhoea. Women who have these symptoms or develop them with an IUD may be suitable for the progestogen IUS.

Barrier methods

These methods are increasingly reliable in this age group as fertility is waning but such methods still demand careful and consistent use. They may be less acceptable as a new option for couples who have used other non-coitus-related methods in the past and for older men who may have increasing erectile dysfunction and may find male condoms exacerbate this.

Condoms also provide protection against sexually transmitted infections (STIs). People of any age entering a new relationship or having several changes of sexual partner are at risk of STIs. The incidence of STIs is rising in all age groups and the contraceptive consultation may be an opportunity to raise awareness of this.

Natural family planning may become more challenging in this age group as periods become irregular in some, and some cycles become anovulatory. The Billings method can be learned from trained counsellors in this method and, provided there is commitment to making the method work, it can be very successful.

Emergency contraception is an important part of the contraceptive package on offer. Many women in their 40s assume that they are relatively infertile but would view a pregnancy as a disaster. Emergency pills were not so widely available when this age group were in their teens and women may not be aware of their efficacy, time scale and low incidence of side effects. Emergency contraception is available free from GPs, contraceptive clinics and genitourinary medicine clinics. It is also available from some community pharmacies; a charge is made for advice and supplies, but this may be less of a deterrent for an older woman than for a teenager, and the anonymity of the pharmacy may appeal.

Sterilization
Male and female sterilization has been discussed. It is important that women are aware of the operative risks from laparoscopy and the fact that female sterilization will not improve menstrual problems. With naturally reduced fertility, methods such as the POP may be recommended as effective contraception, avoiding the operative risks of sterilization.

Women have different priorities when it comes to contraception, and the choice a woman makes will be different at different stages in her life. Factors such as chronic illness, smoking, weight, menstrual irregularities and belief systems must be taken into account when discussing contraceptive options.

Further reading

Davies L. Access by the unaccompanied under-16-year-old adolescent to general practice without parental consent. J Fam Plann Reprod Health Care 2003;29(4):205–7.
Faculty of Family Planning, www.ffprhc.org (for guidelines).
Guillebaud J. Contraception: your questions answered. Churchill Livingstone; London, 2003.
Royal College of General Practitioners and Brook. Confidentiality and Young People: improving teenagers' uptake of sexual and other health care advice. A toolkit for general practice, primary care groups and trusts. RCGP: London, 2000.

Dysuria and urethral discharge in men

Steve Baguley

It is very unusual for a woman to complain specifically of urethral discharge and if a woman reports dysuria it is usually due to a urinary tract infection. Only rarely does chlamydia cause dysuria in women. However, urethritis due to an STI should always be suspected in a man who complains of these symptoms.

History

- Ask about the onset of symptoms and any associated problems, e.g. ulceration on the outside of the penis might indicate that there could also be ulcers in the urethra.
- Have any of his sexual partners recently been diagnosed with anything?
- Scrotal contents pain might be due to epididymo-orchitis; if this is confirmed on examination it would necessitate different treatment from an uncomplicated urethritis.
- Ask about other urinary symptoms such as frequency, urgency or haematuria, which could indicate that this is a urinary tract infection (UTI) after all.
- Has he had any STIs before? If a partner was not treated last time, he could have the same one back again.
- A sexual history is essential, although do not rule out an STI just because his history is low risk. Remember that most STIs can be acquired through oral sex too.
- Ask about drug treatment. Has he taken any antibiotics for the problem, either prescribed or bought over the counter, as is possible in South East Asia and other regions. Note any drug allergies.

Examination

- Initial examination is best performed with the patient standing, since this enables easy examination of the scrotal contents. Some clinicians feel uncomfortable having a semi-naked man standing in front of them and prefer the patient to sit or lie on a couch.
- Check for inguinal lymphadenopathy. If found, this could be a clue toward a diagnosis of herpes, even if no ulceration is seen on further examination.
- Lymphadenopathy is very unusual in chlamydial or gonorrhoeal urethritis. If found, this should raise suspicions of lymphogranuloma venereum (see page 141)
- Examine the scrotal contents. This is a good opportunity to discuss the importance of testicular self-examination. Check for swelling and/or tenderness

of the epididymi and the testes themselves. Interpreted in conjunction with the sexual history, such signs could indicate the need to treat for epididymitis (see page 99).

- Look for ulceration or blistering of the genital skin. Even in a first episode of genital herpes, such signs could be very mild. If herpes is healing you might just see a small area of scabbed skin.
- If the man is uncircumcized, ask him to pull back his foreskin or do it yourself. A penile discharge might actually be caused by a problem under the foreskin such as a malignancy. Other causes of a subpreputial discharge include anaerobic balanitis and certain dermatoses such as erosive lichen planus (see page 109).
- Next look at the urethral meatus. There might be an obvious urethral discharge but if not, milk the urethra to try and elicit one. This is best done by holding the penis in one hand and placing the index finger of the other hand over the urethra on the underside of the penis just in front of the scrotum. If you then move your finger forward on the urethra, this can squeeze discharge forward to appear at the meatus.
- If you see an obvious yellow/greenish discharge, it is almost certainly gonorrhoea (and maybe chlamydia too). If you see a clear discharge it is probably not gonorrhoea but could be chlamydia or another cause of urethritis.

Tests

The main conditions one needs to consider in a man presenting with symptoms of urethritis are chlamydia (page 93) and gonorrhoea (page 114). A large number of other conditions can also cause urethritis (NSU, page 146), although tests for most of them are not widely available.

Which tests you do depends on the setting you are working in and the facilities you have available. Although all sexual health clinics will test for chlamydia and gonorrhoea, the specimens and tests used vary round the world. The most likely specimens and tests would be:

- one urethral swab, which is used for:
  - preparing a slide for Gram-stained microscopy
  - inoculating an agar plate for gonorrhoea culture
  - a nucleic acid amplification test (e.g. polymerase chain reaction (PCR) or strand displacement amplification (SDA)).
- or one urethral swab and a 20-ml first-void urine sample, which are used for:
  - preparing a slide for Gram-stained microscopy (swab)
  - gonorrhoea culture (direct plating as above or sent to lab in charcoal transport medium) (swab)
  - chlamydia nucleic acid amplification test (NAAT) as above or enzyme immunoassay (EIA) (urine).
- or two urethral swabs, which are used for:
  - preparing a slide for Gram-stained microscopy (first swab)
  - gonorrhoea culture (direct plating as above or sent to lab) (first swab)
  - chlamydia NAAT or EIA (second swab).

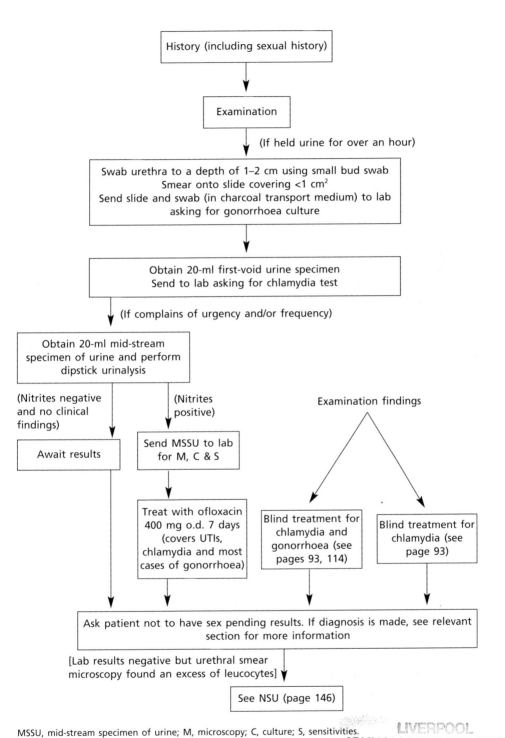

History (including sexual history)

↓

Examination

↓ (If held urine for over an hour)

Swab urethra to a depth of 1–2 cm using small bud swab
Smear onto slide covering <1 cm^2
Send slide and swab (in charcoal transport medium) to lab
asking for gonorrhoea culture

↓

Obtain 20-ml first-void urine specimen
Send to lab asking for chlamydia test

↓ (If complains of urgency and/or frequency)

Obtain 20-ml mid-stream
specimen of urine and perform
dipstick urinalysis

(Nitrites negative
and no clinical
findings)

(Nitrites
positive)

Examination findings

Await results

Send MSSU to lab
for M, C & S

↓

Treat with ofloxacin
400 mg o.d. 7 days
(covers UTIs,
chlamydia and most
cases of gonorrhoea)

Blind treatment for
chlamydia and
gonorrhoea (see
pages 93, 114)

Blind treatment for
chlamydia (see
page 93)

Ask patient not to have sex pending results. If diagnosis is made, see relevant
section for more information

[Lab results negative but urethral smear
microscopy found an excess of leucocytes]

See NSU (page 146)

MSSU, mid-stream specimen of urine; M, microscopy; C, culture; S, sensitivities.

Figure 1 Procedure for a man presenting with discharge or dysuria

Over the next few years, NAAT tests for gonorrhoea will become more widely available in the UK – this will enable testing for chlamydia and gonorrhoea from a single specimen of first-void urine.

If you are working in primary care the tests you use will vary depending on what tests the lab offers.

The flow chart (see Figure 1) gives an outline of what should be done for a man presenting to primary care complaining of discharge or dysuria.

Urethral irritation

If the chlamydia and gonorrhoea tests are negative and the urethral smear microscopy comes back normal, despite the man holding his urine for a prolonged period, then he probably does not have urethritis. Unfortunately, the causes of a sensation of urethral irritation in the absence of inflammation are poorly understood. A variety of conditions/activities are anecdotally thought to be associated with the symptom including:

- neuropathic pain
- chronic pelvic pain
- repeated squeezing of the urethra
- over-enthusiastic masturbation or sexual activity
- concentrated urine caused by dehydration
- alcohol – perhaps more likely the concentrated urine of the following morning
- allergies, e.g. to shower gels used as an aid to masturbation.

The man should be reassured that he does not have a sexually transmitted infection and given appropriate advice depending on the suspected cause.

Genital itch

Venkat Gudi

Genital itch is a common complaint. Although many conditions that cause generalized pruritus can affect the genital area, only conditions in which genital itch is a particular feature are included here. Pruritus ani is excluded from this section since its myriad causes would require more space than is available

History of presenting complaint

- How long has the patient had the problem? Pruritus of short duration is usually related to an infection (for example dermatophyte, candidiasis, scabies or pediculosis pubis) or dermatitis (either irritant or allergic). Chronic pruritus is more commonly related to inflammatory disorders of skin and mucous membranes.
- Is the itch confined to a small part of the genital skin, the whole genital area or does it affect the whole body?
- Are there associated symptoms such as vaginal discharge, rash or ulceration?
- Have they had any significant ill health in the past or any sexually transmitted infections? Ask about skin diseases such as eczema and psoriasis and any history of allergy.
- Take a drug history. Have they tried treating the itch with anything, or could the itching be due to a drug allergy?
- As with any genital complaint, a sexual history (see page 3) is essential. If the history suggests that they could have acquired an STI, offer them an STI screen as well as an assessment of what is causing the itch.

Examination

The best clue to the cause of the itch is to first consider the area that is itchy see Table 1.

Table 1 Clinical features of possible causes of genital itch

Location	Appearance	Diagnoses to consider	Action
Generalized itch but particularly bad in genital region	3–10 mm red, often flaky papules/nodules on scrotum, penile shaft or vulva. Person complaining of generalized itch. Might be a fine macular rash on trunk. Linear scaly appearance on finger webs or inner aspect of wrists.	Scabies	See page 162 for further information and management advice

continued overleaf

Table 1 continued

Location	Appearance	Diagnoses to consider	Action
Any genital site	Fluid-filled blisters or pustules, usually tender, might have tender inguinal lymphadeno-pathy. Often slight redness and swelling around the lesions. Might have flu-like symptoms	Herpes	See page 124 for further information and management advice
	Discrete red patches, usually with central clearing and a rim of scale	Dermatophyte infection	Ideally skin scrapings should be sent to the microbiology laboratory for fungal studies before starting treatment. Try an azole antifungal with a mild steroid, e.g. Daktarin HC cream b.d. for 4 weeks. If symptoms return follow-ing blind treatment, send skin scrapings for fungal microscopy and culture
	Thickened white skin with accentuated skin markings, usually seen on vulva but also on scrotum. Less common on penis	Lichen simplex	See page 103 for further information and management advice
	Discrete red patches. Surface scale unusual. Mild itch only. Might have similar albeit scalier lesions in other sites such as back of the elbows	Psoriasis	See page 106 for further information and management advice
	No obvious rash.	Iron deficiency, hypothyroidism, hepatic or renal impairment. Psychological	Full blood count, ferritin, thyroid status and serum biochemistry. Consider referral to psychologist if all other tests negative.
	Skin red in folds, particularly perianal region in children. Apparently superinfected genital dermatosis	Beta-haemolytic streptococci, coliforms or Staphylococcus aureus cellulitis	Swab for bacteriology to identify the causal organism, and discover antibiotic sensitivity profile
Pubic hair	1-mm diameter dark brown dots adherent to hairs and/or 2-mm diameter pale brown insects gripping tightly to skin. Might complain of having black specks (dried blood) appearing in underwear	Pubic lice, aka crab lice	See page 149 for further information and management advice
Vulva	Thick white discharge visible externally or on speculum examination. Sometimes reddening of vulval skin and	Vulvovaginal candidosis, aka thrush	See page 184 for further information and management advice

	fissuring, particularly around perineum		
	Thin discharge, sometimes seems frothy when examined with a speculum. Sometimes reddening of vulval skin extending to thighs	Trichomoniasis	See page 181 for further information and management advice
	White areas of thinned skin probably containing small ecchymoses (bleeding into skin)	Lichen sclerosus. This also occurs in men, but itch is not a prominent feature for men	See page 107 for further information and management advice
	Flat warty area, poorly responsive to standard wart treatment. Might be pigmented. Patient might have a history of cervical intraepithelial neoplasia (CIN) and probably smokes	Vulval intraepithelial neoplasia	Refer to vulval clinic if available. Otherwise refer to colposcopy.
Groin	Characteristically, central clearing and peripheral scaling are seen in annular lesions. Darkened skin is seen in chronic disease	Tinea cruris (a dermatophyte infection)	Good hygiene important – wash with plain water and dry well. Try an azole antifungal with a mild steroid, e.g. Daktarin HC cream b.d. for 4-6 weeks
Uncircumcised glans penis	Red blotchy rash	Balanitis (not a diagnosis in its own right. It's a sign of a large, disparate group of conditions)	Good hygiene important – wash with plain water and dry well. Try an azole antifungal with a mild steroid, e.g. Daktarin HC cream b.d. for 2 weeks

Hopefully by now you have made a diagnosis and decided on treatment or referral. If in doubt, refer to a GUM physician or dermatologist. Some hospitals have special clinics for penile or vulval dermatology staffed by specialists from both departments (and often a gynaecologist or urologist).

General advice for anogenital pruritus includes avoidance of moisture, careful drying if wet, wearing white cotton instead of synthetic undergarments, avoiding prolonged seating on vinyl surfaces to reduce sweating, as well as avoidance of perfumed products or coloured wipes (to decrease the risk of contact sensitization). An emollient such as diprobase or aqueous cream should be used as a soap substitute. Patch testing may be helpful in a few patients, especially if there is any associated erythema. It is preferable to use ointments instead of creams for topical treatment in the anogenital region, as the latter generally contain preservatives and are likely to cause contact allergy.

If you think that the itch is due to an STI, then as well as offering the appropriate treatment it is important to recommend tests for other infections that could have been acquired during the same encounter.

Further reading

Weichert GE. An approach to the treatment of anogenital pruritus. Dermatol Ther 2004; 17(1):129–33.

Genital skin lumps

Steve Baguley

Noticing a lump on the anogenital skin is a common reason for people to attend a genitourinary medicine clinic. The person might be convinced that the lump is new, but it is often the case that the lump has been there for some time and for some reason the person has only recently become aware of it.

History of presenting complaint

> • Clarify what they mean by a 'lump', some people might describe something that sounds more like an ulcer.
> • Where exactly is the lump?
> • How long has it been there?
> • Are there any associated symptoms such as pain, itching or bleeding?
> • Do they have any symptoms elsewhere such as generalized itch?
> • Have they had any significant ill health in the past or any sexually transmitted infections?
> • Take a drug history. Have they tried treating the lump with anything?

As with any genital complaint, a sexual history (page 3) is essential. This might reveal that the lump could be due to an STI but you could find that the person has never had sexual contact. The history might give you a clue as to why the person has only just noticed the lump – guilt or anxiety about a sexual encounter is a common reason for people starting to pay more attention to their genitals.

If the history suggests that they could have acquired an STI, offer them an STI screen.

Examination

The lump might be immediately obvious but, if it is not, ask the person to point it out to you. See Table 1 for the clinical features of various types of genital skin lumps.

Table 1 Clinical features of genital skin lumps

Normal or sexually acquired	Appearance	Probable cause	Action
Normal findings or variants	1-mm-diameter smooth pale papules, sometimes filiform, in a ring around the penile corona	Coronal papillae, aka penile pearly papules	Explain that they are normal and that no treatment is needed

continued

Table 1 continued

Normal or sexually acquired	Appearance	Probable cause	Action
	1-mm-diameter smooth whitish papules either side of the penile frenulum, usually symmetrical	Tyson's glands: modified sebaceous glands	Explain that they are normal and that no treatment is needed
	Pale, yellowish punctate appearance under the skin surface, made more obvious by stretching the skin. Usually seen on the underside of the foreskin or the labia minora	Fordyce spots: sebaceous glands	Explain that they are normal and that no treatment is needed
	Filiform surface on lateral sides of vaginal introitus, usually flesh coloured	Vulval papillomatosis	Explain that this is normal and that no treatment is needed
	Pale, often yellowish papules usually 2–3 mm across but can be up to 10 mm. Most common on scrotum and penile shaft but also seen on labia majora	Sebaceous glands. If larger, they have probably hyper-trophied as a result of being picked or have become infected	They are normal and should not be picked
	Soft, smooth fleshy tissue at the inner margin of the vulvar vestibule	Hymenal remnants	Explain that this is normal and that no treatment is needed
Probably sexually acquired	3–10 mm, red, often flaky papules/nodules on scrotum, penile shaft or vulva. Person complaining of generalized itch. Might be a fine macular rash on trunk. Linear scaly appearance on finger webs or inner aspect of wrists	Scabies	See page 162 for further information and management advice
	Roughened papules, often slightly paler than surrounding skin. Found anywhere in anogenital region but common at posterior fourchette (the side of the vagina closest to the perineum) and around the foreskin. Also seen in the urethral meatus and perianally. On thin mucosa, the capillary pattern can be seen within them. Vary in size from barely visible to a few centimetres across	Anogenital warts	See page 187 for further information and management advice
	Smooth papules, often with a central depression (hard to see on small ones). Seen anywhere on anogenital skin, including lower abdomen and pubic area. Usually 2–8 mm in diameter, occasionally bigger if patient is immunosuppressed	Molluscum contagiosum	See page 144 for further information and management advice

continued overleaf

Table 1 continued

Normal or sexually acquired	Appearance	Probable cause	Action
	Hard fleshy lesions in perianal area or vaginal introitus. Risk group for syphilis, e.g. contact with someone from a country where syphilis is common, or men who have sex with men (MSM). Probably has a macular rash elsewhere on body	Condylomata lata. A sign of secondary syphilis	See page 106 for further information and management advice
	Fluid-filled blisters or pustules, usually tender, might have tender inguinal lymphadenopathy. Often slight redness and swelling around the lesions. Might have flu-like symptoms	Herpes	See page 124 for further information and management advice
Other conditions	Usually solitary subcutaneous nodule, flesh-coloured unless infected. Seen anywhere except subpreputially and in the vaginal introitus	Epidermoid cyst, aka sebaceous cyst	Usually best left alone. If enucleated by squeezing, the material simply reaccumulates. If large and inconvenient, they can be surgically removed. If infected, antibiotics, e.g. flucloxacillin 500 mg q.i.d. 7 days (unless penicillin allergic), can reduce inflammation
	Roughened papules, usually slightly darker than surrounding skin. Found almost anywhere on body. Not usually seen sub-preputially or in the vaginal introitus. More common in older people. Usually have a slightly greasy surface (though this is hard to feel when wearing gloves!)	Basal cell papilloma, aka sebaceous wart	Can be left untreated. If treatment required for cosmetic reasons or due to concern that it is a viral wart, cryotherapy is effective
	Indurated, erythematous skin with pustules. Some-times inguinal lymphadeno-pathy. Seen anywhere	Furunculosis	Swab pustules. Often requires systemic anti-biotics. Usually caused by S. aureus so try flucloxacillin 500 mg q.i.d. 7 days (unless penicillin allergic)
	Pustules at hair follicles. Seen in any site. In genital area usually seen in pubic region	Folliculitis	Topical antiseptic or antibiotic (e.g. mupirocin ointment) usually adequate
	1–2 mm, red maculopapules usually seen on scrotum. Non-tender	Angiokeratomata	No treatment needed.

Hopefully by now you have made a diagnosis and decided on treatment or referral. If in doubt refer to a GUM physician or dermatologist. Some hospitals have special clinics for penile or vulval dermatology staffed by specialists from both departments (and often a gynaecologist or urologist).

If you find that the lump is a normal variant, you might be able to relate the patient's concern to an episode in their history such as sex outside a long-term relationship that has made them concerned about STIs. If you think that the lump is due to an STI, then as well as offering the appropriate treatment it is important to recommend tests for other infections that could have been acquired from the same encounter.

Genital ulceration

Andrew Leung

Introduction

Genital ulceration is defined as lesions characterized by the loss of epithelium in the skin or mucosa of the genital area. A regional lymphadenopathy often accompanies the ulceration. The combination of ulceration and lymphadenopathy constitutes the genital ulcer adenopathy syndrome. The importance of genital ulcer disease has increased considerably since it became evident that these lesions may increase the risk of HIV transmission.

Genital ulcers are more common in developing countries than in the developed world. In Europe and North America, 1–5% of STI patients present with genital ulceration, whereas the comparable figure for Africa and Asia is 20–70%. The aetiology of genital ulceration also shows remarkable geographic variability. Genital herpes (page 124) is by far the most frequent cause in Europe and North America, whereas chancroid (page 90) is more common in sub-Saharan Africa and South East Asia. Lymphogranuloma venereum (LGV) (page 141) is endemic in parts of Africa, India, South America, the Caribbean and parts of South East Asia. Donovanosis (page 97) is largely restricted to Papua New Guinea, southern Africa, north-east Brazil, French Guyana and the aboriginal communities in northern Australia.

Aetiology

The most frequent infectious causes of genital ulceration are herpes simplex virus (HSV) (genital herpes), *Treponema pallidum* (syphilis), *Haemophilus ducreyi* (chancroid), the L-serovars of *Chlamydia trachomatis* (LGV) and *Klebsiella granulomatis* (donovanosis). Other causes include Behçet's and Reiter's syndromes (page 165), fixed drug eruption, erythema multiforme, Crohn's disease, aphthous ulcers, erosive lichen planus (page 109), trauma, candidiasis and malignancy.

Clinical features

The classical presentation of genital ulceration often does not correspond to the textbook descriptions. Diagnosis is sometimes difficult because clinical presentations are often atypical and mixed infections are common, especially in developing countries. In addition, secondary bacterial or fungal infections, application of antibiotics or corticosteroids and the presence of immunodeficiency as in HIV disease, can alter the clinical appearance of ulcers.

History

A medical history with a detailed sexual history is essential in determining the likely aetiology of genital ulcers. The likelihood of an infectious cause increases if there has been a recent change of sexual partner. Place of origin, ethnic group and foreign travel may suggest an increased risk of certain diseases (e.g. chancroid, LGV and donovanosis). Most cases of syphilis and LGV diagnosed in Europe in the past few years have been in men who have sex with men. A drug and allergy history may indicate fixed drug eruption or erythema multiforme.

The sexual history may help to identify the infection source and hence the incubation period. In general, the incubation periods for chancroid (1–14 days) and genital herpes (2–20 days) are short, whereas they are usually longer for syphilis (9–90 days), LGV (3 days to 6 weeks) and donovanosis (1–4 weeks, but up to 6 months). However, it is not always easy to identify the correct source of the infection, especially if there are multiple partners or if long incubation periods are involved. Unlike infectious ulcerations, which have incubation periods of days to weeks, traumatic ulcers usually develop quickly (within 24 hours) after the causative effect.

Pain is not a universal symptom in genital ulceration. Whereas ulcers in genital herpes, chancroid and Behçet's are generally painful, those in syphilis and LGV are usually painless. Donovanosis ulcers are either painless or only mildly painful.

Another important question in the history is whether or not the ulcers are restricted to the genital area. Ulceration involving both genital and non-genital sites suggests non-venereal origin such as Behçet's, erythema multiforme, lichen planus or aphthous ulcers. In Crohn's disease, the ulcers are normally associated with symptoms of bowel disease.

Examination
A presumptive diagnosis can sometimes be made by the characteristic appearance of the ulcers, their distribution and associated findings. However, these characteristics are often atypical as a result of secondary infections and mixed aetiologies. Most genital ulcers in men are found on the penile shaft, the prepuce, near the frenulum and in the coronal sulcus. In women, lesions may occur on the labia, fourchette, vagina, cervix and perianal area. Typically, the lesions of primary syphilis and LGV are solitary, whereas those of genital herpes, chancroid and donovanosis are multiple.

In genital herpes, small clusters of vesicles on an erythematous base first appear and these soon develop into multiple shallow ulcers. In syphilis, the papule develops into an ulcer with a sharply demarcated and raised edge. The base is smooth and non-purulent. In chancroid, the papules surrounded by erythema become pustules. These in turn rupture to form ulcers with ragged, undermined and irregular edges. The base has yellow-grey exudates and bleeds easily. In LGV, the small ulcers with elevated and oval edges heal quickly and often go unnoticed. In donovanosis, the lesion is indolent and progressive with a 'beefy' red base and granulation-like tissue. In Behçet's syndrome, the lesions begin as small papules that erode to form erythematous, punched-out ulcers. In Crohn's disease, the ulcers are often described as deep and knife-cut.

When present, features of the associated regional lymphadenopathy may also be helpful in differentiating the different aetiologies. These include their consistency, tenderness, fluctuance and whether they are bilateral or unilateral. The lymphadenopathy in primary syphilis is usually discrete, bilateral, firm and painless, whereas those in genital herpes are also often bilateral but are usually smaller and tender. In contrast, the lymphadenopathy associated in either chancroid or LGV is usually unilateral and tender. It may also undergo suppuration to form inguinal abscesses (buboes) and rupture. LGV usually involves several nodes, and when both inguinal and femoral nodes are swollen and divided by the inguinal ligament, this creates the classic 'groove-sign'. The pseudobuboes in donovanosis are not due to infected lymph nodes; they are granulomatous nodules in the subcutaneous tissue of the inguinal region.

Laboratory diagnosis

A good clinical history and a thorough physical examination provide useful indications to the aetiology of the genital lesions, and can often lead to a presumptive diagnosis. In order to obtain a definitive diagnosis of genital ulceration, laboratory evaluation should be performed.

Collection of specimens

For dark-ground microscopy (diagnosis of primary syphilis), the ulcer should be washed with saline and dried with gauze. It is then squeezed between thumb and index finger until an exudate appears. This exudate should then be collected by a loop or a cover slip.

Specimens for HSV culture are best obtained following disruption of vesicles and collection of vesicle fluid. If lesions are already ulcerated, the specimen is collected by swabbing of the base of the ulcer. Swabbing the ulcer base also provides specimens for cultures of *H. ducreyi* and *C. trachomatis*. In cases of suspected donovanosis, materials are used from scrapings obtained from the edges of the lesions or from punch biopsy. Biopsy is also indicated in atypical ulcers, in ulcers of suspected non-infectious causes (e.g. Behçet's and Crohn's) and in cases of suspected malignancy.

When fluctuant lymph nodes (buboes) are present, needle aspiration provides specimens for cultures of *C. trachomatis* and *H. ducreyi* and for dark-ground microscopy to exclude *T. pallidum*.

Blood is collected for serological tests for syphilis and LGV.

Microscopy

Dark-ground microscopic examination remains the gold standard for diagnosis of early syphilis. The organism *T. pallidum* is recognised by its morphology and characteristic movement. However, the procedure requires a suitably adapted microscope and considerable technical expertise to discriminate between *T. pallidum* and other spirochetes. In chancroid, direct examination of the specimen by a Gram stain may reveal pleomorphic Gram-negative organisms in a 'school of fish' pattern. However, interpretation is often difficult and the test is not reliable.

In genital herpes, antigen can be detected by using immunofluorescence. However, sensitivity of this test is low and viral culture remains the method of choice. In donovanosis, diagnosis is dependent upon the demonstration of intracytoplasmic encapsulated Donovan bodies within mononuclear cells in Giemsa- or Wright-stained smears.

Culture

Viral culture is the method of choice for the diagnosis of genital herpes. Isolation of *H. ducreyi* from a genital ulcer or lymph node provides a definitive diagnosis of chancroid.

However, culture of *H. ducreyi* is difficult and may not be offered by all laboratories. It is important to request culture media from the laboratory in advance so the specimen can be plated immediately after collection. Gonococcal agar base supplemented with bovine haemoglobin, foetal calf serum and vancomycin is often used.

Formerly, culture of chlamydia from lesional material was used for diagnosing LGV but its low sensitivity and limited availability is making NAAT testing more popular.

Serology

All patients with genital ulceration should have serological tests for syphilis. They may be negative when the patient presents with a chancre, but will usually become positive during secondary syphilis. Serological tests should not replace dark-ground microscopy in the diagnosis of primary syphilis, but could be used to further evaluate genital ulcers and to quantify response to treatment.

Serology is rarely useful in the diagnosis of primary herpes. In LGV, the chlamydial complement-fixation test, which measures antibody to chlamydial group antigen, is the most widely used serological test although is not specific for the L serovars.

Molecular techniques

The development of amplification techniques such as the polymerase chain reaction (PCR) has resulted in methods that are both sensitive and specific to the detection of the organisms associated with genital ulceration. They are, however, expensive, requiring special containment laboratories, appropriate equipment and expert staff. PCR is becoming widely used for the detection of HSV and has also been used (mainly in research) to detect the presence of *T. pallidum* and *H. ducreyi*. A multiplex PCR has also been developed to detect the presence of these three organisms in a single ulcer specimen.

Nucleic acid amplification tests for *C. trachomatis* such as PCR and strand displacement amplification give a positive result when testing for the L serovars that cause LGV. However, further molecular tests are necessary to say precisely which serovar is involved.

Management (For the management of specific conditions, see the relevant sections.)

With the exception of genital herpes, treatment is normally initiated after establishment of a definitive laboratory diagnosis. In the case of primary genital herpes, appropriate antiviral therapy should be commenced at the time of clinical diagnosis. In settings where laboratory support is limited and mixed infections are common, syndromic management can be initiated. This approach is recommended by the World Health Organisation (WHO), particularly for developing countries. With the exception of *H. ducreyi,* antimicrobial resistance is not yet a major problem.

In ulcers where secondary bacterial infections are present, treatment may consist simply of frequent application of warm-water compresses to remove necrotic material and purulent exudates. In severe cases, a broad-spectrum antibiotic should be given. Until syphilis can be definitely excluded, a non-treponemicidal antimicrobial such as cotrimoxazole should be used. The fluctuant buboes of LGV and chancroid should be aspirated through adjacent healthy skin to avoid fistula formation.

In fixed drug eruption and in erythema multiforme, the offending medication should be discontinued immediately. Topical corticosteroids should not be used in infectious ulcers but are useful in lichen planus, aphthous ulcers and mild Behçet's syndrome. Systemic corticosteroids may be required in erythema multiforme and in Crohn's disease.

Haematospermia

Sunil Kumar and Raj Persad

Haematospermia is an alarming symptom and is defined as the presence of blood in the seminal fluid.

Causes of haematospermia

- inflammation of the prostate, urethra and seminal vesicles
- prostatic calculi
- prostate cancer
- post-transrectal ultrasound and biopsy of the prostate
- infections (e.g.) tuberculosis
- seminal vesicle abnormalities.

Evaluation

Patients have to be reassured as most of the time there is no underlying pathology, but prostate cancer should be ruled out – particularly in the over 50s. Haematospermia usually takes several weeks to resolve. If it is persistent or recurrent then the patient should be investigated for

- coagulopathies
- hypertension
- prostate cancer [rectal examination and prostate specific antigen (PSA) should be performed to exclude prostate cancer]
- congenital or acquired anomalies. Transrectal ultrasound (TRUS) to look for seminal vesicle abnormalities, prostatic calculi and ejaculatory duct pathology should be performed. Only rarely may cystoscopy be useful.

Haematospermia nearly always resolves spontaneously and the patient should be warned that it might take several months and several ejaculations to clear. Treatment is otherwise aimed at the underlying cause such as appropriate antibiotics for prostatitis or the surgical excision of seminal vesicle cysts or calculi.

Further reading

Ganabathi K, Chadwick D, Feneley RC, Gingell JC. Haematospermia (review). Br J Urol 1992; 69(3):225–30.

Haematuria

Sunil Kumar and Raj Persad

Blood in the urine (haematuria) can be a very distressing symptom and can be either microscopic or macroscopic. Urine containing more than three red blood cells/high-power field should be regarded as at least microscopic haematuria. It is essential to differentiate between haematuria of renal origin and that of urological origin. Haematuria of renal origin is usually associated with proteinuria and urine microscopy will demonstrate the presence of casts. In the presence of proteinuria, the patient should be referred to a renal physician and further investigations should include creatinine, 24-hour urinary protein assessment and creatinine clearance. Under renal physician advice, possibly a renal biopsy may also be required. The most important urological cause of haematuria to exclude is that of urinary tract malignancy, but there are other important non-malignant conditions that may need urgent attention such as urinary tract stones (see below).

False positives – In women, menstrual history is important as the specimen can get contaminated and yield a false-positive result. False positive results can also occur after physical exertion and dehydration. Conditions such as haemoglobinuria and myoglobinuria should be excluded. Urine dipsticks have over 90% sensitivity in picking up microscopic haematuria.

It is important to note that frank haematuria generally resolves spontaneously, but a small group of patients may require admission as they present with clot retention.

Common causes of haematuria

- urinary tract infections
- calculus disease
- transitional cell carcinoma of the urinary tract
- renal cell cancer
- intrinsic renal disease (e.g.) nephropathies
- polycystic kidney disease
- renal artery/vein thrombosis
- renal trauma
- arteriovenous (AV) fistula
- coagulation disorders
- papillary necrosis.

Evaluation

History forms an important aspect of haematuria evaluation. Information on cigarette smoking and occupational history are essential as there is a link between transitional cell carcinoma of the urinary tract and exposure to certain chemicals. Physical examination should include abdominal examination to look for masses and a rectal examination to rule out associated prostate cancer. Urinalysis should include microscopy, culture and sensitivity. Urine should also be sent for cytology to look for frankly malignant cells or atypical cells, which may indicate an underlying malignancy. Cytology is also useful to diagnose carcinoma in situ and for follow-up purposes. It is not useful in the presence of frank haematuria in the specimen.

Ultrasound of the urinary tract is an essential investigation and usually picks up any abnormalities in the kidneys. Sometimes abnormalities of the bladder can also be visualized, but flexible cystoscopy is more sensitive in diagnosing bladder lesions. In the presence of active haematuria, flexible cystoscopy is not useful as visualization is poor. It is therefore essential for the haematuria to settle prior to the cystoscopy. An intravenous urogram (IVU) completes the investigation cycle for haematuria and is more sensitive in picking up ureteric tumours that the ultrasound may have missed (Table 1).

Recommendations

Table 1 Recommended tests for patients with haematuria

	Men over 40 and women over 50	Men under 40 and women under 50
Microscopic haematuria	Renal ultrasound, flexible cystoscopy and an IVU if there are risk factors	No need to investigate unless there are obvious risk factors
Macroscopic haematuria	Renal ultrasound, flexible cystoscopy and an IVU if required	Renal ultrasound, flexible cystoscopy and an IVU if required

Further reading

Gillatt DA, O'Reilly PH. Haematuria analysed – a prospective study. J R Soc Med 1987; 80(9):559–60.

Khadra MH, Pickard RS, Charlton M et al. A prospective analysis of 1930 patients with haematuria to evaluate current diagnostic practice. J Urol 2000;163(2):524–7.

Incontinence

Sunil Kumar and Raj Persad

Urinary incontinence is defined as any involuntary leakage of urine. **Stress incontinence** is the commonest form and is the involuntary loss of urine on physical exertion when the rise in intra-abdominal pressure overcomes the continent forces of the internal and external urethral sphincter mechanisms.

Risk factors for stress incontinence

- constitutional – more common in:
  - caucasians
  - the obese
  - women
  - the elderly
- urogynaecological
  - cystocoele
  - prolapse
  - hysterectomy
  - previous pelvic surgery
  - oestrogen deficiency
  - pregnancy
- behavioural
  - caffeine, alcohol and tobacco consumption
  - low physical activity
  - poor bladder (and pelvic floor) training
  - constipation
  - bowel dysfunction

Evaluation

Physical examination is important to assess the degree of incontinence and associated conditions and to assess the integrity of the pelvic floor. It is also necessary to note the presence of any coexistent cystocoele or rectocoele. Urodynamic evaluation should be performed if operative intervention is to be considered.

Treatment

Conservative treatment:
- pelvic floor exercises
- tablet therapy (e.g. agents that increase sphincteric tone such as duloxetine)

- vaginal weights
- weight loss and control of chronic cough or asthma.

Surgical intervention:
- injectables with collagen and Macroplastique to 'bulk up' or create urethral 'cushions' internally
- sling procedures (e.g. transvaginal or transobturator tape procedures) to 'tighten' or obstruct the outflow tract minimally invasively
- colposuspension (open surgery to do the same as slings, essentially)
- associated anterior and posterior vaginal wall repairs
- artificial urinary sphincter insertion – these prosthetic devices are expensive and may be prone to failure over time as well as infection.

Urge incontinence

This is defined as the sudden loss of urine preceded by a strong urge to void. It can be seen in patients with cystitis, neurogenic bladders, bladder outflow obstruction, idiopathic detrusor overactivity and interstitial cystitis. Urge incontinence may be secondary to an underlying pathology, which if identified and treated, will usually lead to symptomatic resolution.

Evaluation

Urinalysis should be undertaken to exclude urinary infection, which may be causing urgency symptoms. A full history and examination is essential, particularly a neurological assessment, as overactive bladder symptoms may occur with neurological conditions such as multiple sclerosis, spinal cord lesions and cerebrovascular events. Assessment of bladder outflow symptoms may give an indication of whether urgency is secondary to obstruction (e.g. urethral stricture, bladder neck obstruction or benign prostatic enlargement). A frequency–volume chart may be useful in assessing the severity of the degree of urgency and/or urge incontinence.

Treatment
A simple trial of bladder retraining with supportive pharmacotherapy in the form of anticholinergics (e.g. oxybutynin, tolterodine, trospium, propiverine or solifenacin) are warranted in the first instance if urgency is the only symptom. Additional conservative measures include restriction of caffeinated drinks, weight loss and bowel function improvement.
For mixed stress and urge incontinence, formal urodynamic testing may be necessary before implementing treatment, however. If conservative measures and pharmacotherapy do not work, further conservative options are limited but may include the administration of intravesical botulinum toxin injections. If all attempts at treatment fail, then major surgery in the form of a bladder augmentation is the definitive surgical treatment with a high success rate. By augmenting the bladder with small bowel, high-pressure unstable bladder contractions are dissipated; however, there are potential quality-of-life implications following this procedure, including production of

mucus, recurrent urinary tract infections and the potential need for self-catheterization of the new 'low-pressure' bladder.

Where urgency is secondary to obstruction, surgical correction is appropriate, e.g.
urethrotomy, or transurethral prostatectomy for an enlarged prostate.

Chronic retention

Where incontinence is due to chronic obstruction, even following removal of the
obstruction, the bladder may not empty properly. Overflow may occur and is characterized by occasional small dribbles of urine and episodes of nocturnal incontinence.
In this situation, the bladder may need to be encouraged to empty more efficiently
by the use of self-catheterization.

Continuous incontinence is rare but may be seen in the presence of vesicovaginal
or ureterovaginal fistulae. Ectopic ureter with the ureteric opening distal to the external urethral sphincter mechanism is an even rarer cause of continuous incontinence.

Further reading

Burgard EC, Fraser MO, Karicheti V et al. New pharmacological treatments for urinary incon-
    tinence and overactive bladder. Curr Opin Investig Drugs 2005;6(1):81–9.
Christofi N, Hextall A. Which procedure for incontinence? J Br Menopause Soc 2005;
    11(1):23–7.
Smith J, Persad R, Smith P, Winder A. Keeping Control: A practical guide to the treatment
    and prevention of female incontinence. Vermillion Press: London, 2001.

Scrotal swellings

Sunil Kumar and Raj Persad

The most important finding to elicit about a swelling arising from the scrotum is whether on examination it is possible to get above the swelling. This is critical in differentiating a scrotal swelling from an inguinoscrotal swelling. Common causes of scrotal swellings are hydrocoele, epididymal cyst, varicocoele, epididymo-orchitis and testicular tumours. We will cover all the above conditions in this chapter except epididymo-orchitis, which is covered in a separate chapter in this book.

Hydrocoele

A hydrocoele is a collection of fluid within the tunica vaginalis. Hydrocoele can be acquired or congenital; secondary to a patent processus vaginalis (PPV). Acquired hydrocoeles can be idiopathic or secondary to tumour, trauma or infection. The tunica vaginalis normally produces 0.5 ml of fluid per day and the fluid collects because of an imbalance between fluid production and absorption. Hydrocoele usually presents as a painless swelling in the scrotum and it can be unilateral or bilateral. The swelling can become painful or uncomfortable if it gets to be large or in the presence of infection. The onset may be gradual or sudden, and one must always be suspicious of an underlying testicular tumour in sudden-onset cases, especially when the testicle is impalpable. Hydrocoeles that decrease in size and reappear later should raise the possibility of a congenital hydrocoele with a PPV, especially in the younger age group.

Examination will usually reveal a scrotal swelling. The testes may be impalpable in a large hydrocoele; if the testis is easily palpable and separate from the swelling, then a diagnosis of an epididymal cyst should be entertained. The swelling is usually fluctuant and transilluminates well, suggesting the presence of clear fluid within the sac. Investigations should include an ultrasound scan if there is concern regarding the underlying testicle and to rule out the possibility of testicular cancer.

Hydrocoele can be managed conservatively if it is asymptomatic and not a cosmetic problem. In patients who have medical co-morbidities and are unfit, aspiration with or without injection of a sclerosing agent such as tetracycline or sodium tetradecyl sulfate can be carried out. This can sometimes lead to infection and the hydrocoele can also recur. Surgical treatment would include ligation of the PPV through an inguinal approach if the hydrocoele is congenital, or incision and drainage of the hydrocoele fluid along with eversion or excision of the tunica vaginalis if the hydrocoele is acquired. Small hydrocoeles can be dealt with by plication of the sac after drainage of the fluid. There is a risk of bleeding with haematoma formation, infection and recurrence of the hydrocoele with any procedure.

Epididymal cyst

This is a cystic swelling arising from the epididymis and usually presents as a painless scrotal swelling. It can become uncomfortable as it enlarges in size. The testis is usually felt as a separate entity from the cyst. An epididymal cyst can also transilluminate well. Conservative management is advised if the cyst is small and asymptomatic. Aspiration is generally not advised, as these cysts are usually multiloculated. If the cyst is large and causing discomfort, surgical excision is usually recommended and the patient is counselled about the possibility of infection, bleeding and recurrence of the cyst.

Varicocoele

Varicocoele is dilatation of the veins of the pampiniform plexus. It is more common on the left side and usually presents with a dragging or aching discomfort in the groin or scrotum. It is important to know that the left testicular vein drains into the left renal vein and therefore varicocoeles on the left side should raise the possibility of a left renal tumour. It is important that all patients with a left varicocoele undergo a renal ultrasound. Varicocoeles usually present with some discomfort and swelling that gets worse during the day and settles at night; this is because the veins engorge during the day as a result of gravity. The enlarged veins feel like a bag of worms on palpation. There is little evidence to suggest that varicocoeles may have a role to play in infertility, although treating the varicocoele may improve seminal parameters, which in turn may help with assisted methods of contraception.

It is reasonable to manage a varicocoele conservatively if the patient is not too bothered by his symptoms. The options of management are either surgical or embolization performed by the radiologist. Surgical options include open surgery, i.e. high (retroperitoneal) or low (inguinal) ligation of the vessels. Laparoscopic ligation of the vessels is also an option. In all these techniques the vas is preserved while the rest of the cord structures are ligated, including the testicular artery. The testes tend to pick up their blood supply from the dartos muscle and the incidence of testicular atrophy is small. Complications of operative intervention are recurrence and the possibility of hydrocoele formation on the ipsilateral side.

Testicular cancer

Any patient aged under 50 years presenting with a swelling arising from the body of the testes should be considered to have a testicular tumour until proven otherwise. Primary neoplasms arising from the testes are germ cell tumours (GCTs). They are classified into seminomas and non-seminomas. Non-seminomas include teratoma, embryonal carcinoma, choriocarcinoma and yolk sac tumours. It is important to know that about 40% of testicular tumours are mixed, having both seminomatous and non-seminomatous elements, and these tumours should really be treated as non-seminomas.

Seminomas have a bimodal distribution with two peak age incidences, one at about 30–40 and the other at about 60 years. Non-seminomatous GCTs have a peak age incidence of between 20 and 30 years. They usually present with a painless scrotal swelling or sometimes with a history of trauma. Occasionally they present with metastatic disease, either with an abdominal mass secondary to para-aortic lymphadenopathy, mediastinal mass and lung or brain metastases. There is a swelling in the body of the testes on examination that is usually hard, craggy and painless. There may be an associated hydrocoele.

An ultrasound of the testes is usually diagnostic. Tumour markers such as α-feto protein (AFP), β human chorionic gonadotrophin (βHCG) and lactic dehydrogenase (LDH) should be checked as soon as the diagnosis is suspected or made. They are not of much diagnostic value, but are extremely important for follow-up purposes. An inguinal orchidectomy is performed to obtain a pathological diagnosis. A scrotal approach is not advocated because of the danger of altering the lymphatic drainage if a scrotal incision is made. Once a diagnosis is made, then staging is commenced in the form of a chest X-ray and CT of the abdomen. The staging system is beyond the scope of this chapter. Seminomas are usually radiosensitive, whereas non-seminomatous GCTs respond to chemotherapy. Sometimes a combination of the two or even surgical excision of metastatic tumour may be required. It is important to remember that the prognosis for patients with these tumours is reasonably good, even if they are metastatic on initial diagnosis.

Further reading

Bullock N, Sibley GN, Whittaker RH. Essential Urology, second edition. Edinburgh: Churchill Livingstone, 1994.

Sexual assault

Tessa Crowley

Throughout history, rape has been regarded as forced sexual intercourse. However, its classification as a crime has varied. Roman law apparently stated that it was a crime that could be committed only against virgins. Cultural and religious beliefs influence the assignment of culpability. In ancient Hebrew law, a married woman could be punished together with her rapist. Today there are still reports from some countries of the 'honour killing' of women who have been raped.

Sexual victimization may give rise to serious sequelae in the victim such as physical injury, infection and psychological problems. It also evokes powerful feelings of disgust and anger within the general population. We want to look after the victim and lock up the assailant, yet at the same time, society judges the person who has been sexually assaulted according to unconscious internal codes. For these reasons, people who have had such experiences often do not want to involve the police. Instead, they might present immediately or after a variable time interval to a variety of health care personnel. First disclosure often occurs within the genitourinary clinic setting when they seek screening for infection.

Definition of terms

The definition of terms used to describe particular types of sexual offences can still vary between countries.

In the UK, the Sexual Offences Act 2003 came into force in May 2004. It introduced new penalties for sex crimes and introduced new offences to make it easier for juries to make fair and balanced decisions on the question of consent. It has redefined 'rape', and created a new offence of 'assault by penetration'. The following are definitions from the Sexual Offences Act 2003.

Rape
A person (*A*) commits an offence if:

- he intentionally penetrates the vagina, anus or mouth of another person (*B*) with his penis
- *B* does not consent to the penetration, and
- *A* does not reasonably believe that *B* consents.

Assault by penetration
A person (*A*) commits an offence if:

- he intentionally penetrates the vagina or anus of another person (*B*) with a part of his body or anything else
- the penetration is sexual
- *B* does not consent to the penetration, and
- *A* does not reasonably believe that *B* consents.

A person convicted of rape or assault by penetration may be imprisoned for life.

Sexual assault

A person (*A*) commits an offence if:

- he intentionally touches another person (*B*)
- the touching is sexual
- *B* does not consent to the touching, and
- *A* does not reasonably believe that *B* consents.

This offence carries a term of imprisonment of up to 10 years.

Incidence

Sexual victimization is under-reported; estimates of risk vary, with some suggesting that the lifetime risk may be as high as one in four for women. The British Crime Survey (BCS) found a 9.7% lifetime risk of any sexual victimization and a 4.9% risk of rape after the age of 16 years. In the year ending March 2003, the total number of sexual offences recorded by police in England and Wales was 48 654 – a 17% rise over the previous year. About 10% of reported sexual assaults are on men.

Risk factors

Society's double sexual standards mean that the woman is often perceived to have been in some way responsible for an attack. Young women who dress fashionably can be seen by some groups as 'leading men on' by being sexually provocative. The woman herself often unconsciously subscribes to this belief system and therefore may believe that her experience was not 'real rape'. This will contribute to the difficulty experienced in coming forward to report the offence.

Risks are highest for women living in inner city or urban areas and from low-income backgrounds.

Studies have shown that young single women between the ages of 16 and 24 are at most risk of sexual victimization, with students more likely to report an incident of sexual victimization. Younger women may be more at risk of acquaintance rape and of being specifically targeted by perpetrators, whereas older women are most affected by partner rape. Partner rape often overlaps with domestic violence, with the woman being caught up in a repetition of sexual and violent attacks. Less than one-third of these women tell anyone at all about the rape. Alcohol, cannabis and other recreational drugs are risk factors in sexual assault. A study in the US found these substances present in the urine of up to 40% of 1179 women victims of sexual assault. A survey of complainants attending a sexual assault referral centre (SARC) in London found that 11% reported recent recreational drug use and 30% had drunk two or more units of alcohol before the assault took place.

Perpetrator

Women are most often sexually assaulted by men they know. The BCS found that most perpetrators were known to their victims in some way, as a friend, acquaintance or family member. It found that current partners were responsible for 45% of the rapes reported and 22% were by acquaintances. Strangers were only responsible for 8% of rapes but 23% of sexual assaults. These findings were not replicated by a London SARC, which reported that strangers or relative strangers had assaulted 52% of the clients seen. It is important to consider that when the victim knows the assailant, there may be fear of reprisals if they report the assault to the police. They may worry that their own family and friends will not believe them. These women often experience multiple incidents of sexual violence.

About three-quarters of reported rape incidents involve verbal threats as well as physical force or violence with a significant risk of physical injury. Partners who assault are most likely to inflict injury. Women are most likely to be raped in their own home, whereas sexual assault occurs more often in a public place.

Penovaginal penetration is the commonest form of assault on women. Anal intercourse is reported in between 6–26% of female complainants, but it is important to remember that there may have been a number of different sexual acts performed by the assailant, including irrumation (forced oral penetration) or cunnilingus.

Less than 7% of reported rapes of a female result in a conviction.

It is important to remember that although rare, women can be perpetrators as well. Women can also be accomplices to luring other unsuspecting victims into traps to be raped by others.

Consequences

Emotional

Rape is a violation of the body and the mind. Each individual responds according to their personal history, previous experience and to the type of assault. There is no one response that can be expected; some people appear to be cut off and controlled, whereas others are overwhelmed with fear, humiliation, guilt and shame. If the assailant is a partner or friend, feelings of betrayal of trust can be a major factor in long-term distress. The person who has been raped may suffer from significant psychological problems afterwards, such as anxiety, fear of being alone, panic attacks, depression, self-harm and suicidal ideation. There can be resulting relationship problems with particular difficulties in terms of sex, with up to 59% having a sexual dysfunction. The most common problem is the avoidance of sex.

Research has shown that post-traumatic stress disorder (PTSD) is the most common post-rape trauma psychopathology. It has been defined by the Diagnostic and Statistical Manual (DSM IV). One study has found that 94% of victims could be classified as suffering from PTSD at 1 week post-assault, with 47% still meeting the criteria at 3 months.

Physical

Physical violence occurs in about 50% of attacks, with studies reporting 31–82% of women having bodily injuries such as contusions, abrasions, choke-related injuries, lacerations and stab or gunshot wounds. Genital injuries have been found in 16–58%; these may range from minor abrasions to severe lacerations or penetrating injuries involving the perineum. The absence of genital injury does not exclude rape.

Pregnancy occurs in about 5% of women of reproductive age. Sexually transmitted infections are found in 4–56% of those screened and reflects the local prevalence. Infection with HIV following rape occurring in the UK is rare but must be considered. Risk of acquisition increases if the rape is of a man, if it is particularly violent or if it occurred in areas defined as high prevalence.

Management

Medical

Following a disclosure of sexual assault, the clinician should establish the following details:

- The time since the assault is important because forensic evidence cannot usually be gathered from the person after 1 week. Screening for sexually transmitted infections should be done ideally at 2 weeks post-assault. Hepatitis vaccination should be started within 3 weeks.
- Have they or do they want to involve the police? If yes, do not continue with the examination.
- Evaluate the relationship of the victim to the assailant and establish any known risk factors with regard to the assailant, if known, such as drug use. Ask whether there was more than one person.
- It is important to establish in a sensitive manner what type of assault took place. If the patient does not want to describe the assault, it may be necessary to ask closed questions such as 'Did he put his penis anywhere else?'
- Take a pre- and post-assault sexual history. This may be relevant if any infection is found.
- Establish risk of pregnancy by exploring current contraception, whether ejaculation occurred and if a condom was used.
- Are there symptoms such as discharge, bleeding, pain etc.
- Offer prophylaxis for common sexually transmitted infections such as chlamydia and gonorrhoea. Instigate rapid hepatitis vaccination if indicated.
- Assess and discuss risk of HIV from this incident. Follow local guidelines if post-exposure prophylaxis (PEP) is indicated. The British Association for Sexual Health and HIV (BASHH) has produced guidelines on the administration of antiretrovirals following potential sexual exposure to HIV.
- Instigate appropriate interventions and investigations for any physical injury.
- Explore what support is available from family or friends and offer what local psychological support is available.
- Establish whether there is any ongoing risk to the patient.

Detailed guidelines for the medical management of sexual assault can be found on the BASHH website

Legal

If the patient wishes to report the assault to the police they will be offered a forensic medical examination by an appropriately trained forensic examiner. The purpose of this is to gather evidence. The type of samples collected depends on the nature of the assault. Consideration must be given to time elapsed since the assault. This can be experienced as another traumatic event, so great care should be taken to allow the patient to feel in control. The examination includes:

- A general examination to look for and document contusions or other injuries. Skin sampling is done if contaminated with bodily fluids. Head or pubic hair is sampled if contaminated. Fingernails are sampled if a history of scratching the assailant is obtained.
- Saliva is collected by swabbing the buccal mucosa and rinsing the mouth with sterile water. Spermatozoa may persist for up to 6–31 hours, and persist longest in the gingival crevices.
- Genital examination is done to look for and document local or internal injury.
- Low and high vaginal swabs and endocervical swabs are taken during speculum examination of the vagina. Spermatozoa may be identified for up to 3–7 days.
- If there has been anal penetration a proctoscopy examination may be performed and internal swabs taken. Spermatozoa have been identified 65 hours after rectal penetration.
- Urine and blood should be obtained for toxicological analysis.

Sexual assault referral centres (SARCs)

SARCs are being developed across the UK and provide supportive and forensically secure environments. Support includes medical management as described above. People who have not involved the police can receive treatment, and if they so choose, can give information anonymously to the police regarding their assault. Forensic evidence can be taken and stored, giving the person time to consider whether they wish to make a complaint. They can access medical follow-up, counselling and support irrespective of police involvement.

It is hoped that in the future there will be one 24-hour national phone number that all people who have been sexually victimized could ring. The aim would be to offer medical evaluations and counselling in order to help that person to find the most appropriate care pathway.

Further reading

British Association for Sexual Health and HIV Guidelines. Management of adult victims of sexual assault. www.BASSH.org
Harne L. J Fam Plann Reprod Health 2002;28(3):120–2.
Lee D. The psychological management of rape and PTSD: clinical issues, assessment and treatment. In: The Psychology of Sexual Health. Miller D, Green J (eds). Blackwell Science: Oxford, 2002.
Myhill A, Allen J. Rape and sexual assault of women: the extent and nature of the problem. British Crime Survey 2002. Home Office Research Study 237. Communication Development Unit. Home Office: London, 2002.
Rogers DJ. Assisting and advising complainants of sexual assault in the family planning setting. J Fam Plann Reprod Health.2002;28(3):127–30.
Saphire Homepage. Improving rape investigation and victim care. www.met.police.uk/sapphire/
Sexual Offences Act 2003. www.legislation.hmso.gov.uk/acts/acts2003/20030042.htm
Wilken J, Welch J. Management of people who have been raped. BMJ 2003;326:458–9.

Transgender patients

Gordon McKenna

Introduction

The purpose of this chapter is to introduce the reader to the concept of gender identity disorder (GID), to give a broad overview of current thoughts on mechanism, to recognize the strengths and weaknesses of the international standard of care (called Harry Benjamin Standards of Care, version 6) and to discuss in broad terms the management of the client group.

It is important to distinguish a number of terms in association with this group of patients.

Gender identity disorder (GID) is a broad term covering all patients who perceive a conflict between their body's physical characteristics and their internalized core sexual identity. Under current psychological teachings, core sexual identity is formed at a very young age, usually around 3 years of age. The conflict arises when this perception of one's own gender is mismatched to the body's external appearance. The onset of puberty only makes this difference worse, and significant psychological distress often ensues. When dissatisfied individuals meet specified criteria in one of two official nomenclatures – the International Classification of Diseases-10 (ICD-10, see Appendix) or the Diagnostic and Statistical Manual of Mental Disorders, Fourth Edition (DSM-IV) – they are formally designated as suffering from a GID. Some persons with GID exceed another threshold – they persistently possess a wish for surgical transformation of their bodies. Not surprisingly, the underlying conflict in itself can give rise to secondary psychological and overtly psychiatric diagnoses. The social consequences cannot be overstated, as society places great emphasis on conforming behaviour appropriate to gender stereotypes.

However, some societies accept the existence of a gender between male and female, e.g. in parts of the South Pacific, where such individuals are thought to be particularly special and are revered. There is thus an implicit difference in this culture in that 'gender discordance' does not necessarily lead to GID.

There is a recognized overlap between transgender patients and transvestite patients, but the two diagnoses are quite separate. Transvestism, or cross-dressing, often for a measure of sexual or emotional gratification, is classified as a paraphilia, but it is recognized that some patients will progress from this over time to consider gender realignment surgery.

The incidence is probably 1 in 30 000 in males and about 1 in 100 000 in females. Higher prevalences have also been reported, and the true figure is speculative. A report from the interdepartmental Working Group on Transsexual People in 2000 estimated that there were around 1300–2000 male-to-female transsexuals and 250–400 female-to-male transsexuals living in the UK. The lobby group Press for Change, however, estimates the number of post-operative transsexuals in the UK to be 5000.

Some authorities strongly believe in a biological basis for GID, with evidence of changes in brain nuclei on imaging and post-mortem studies. Other writers argue that there is a psychodynamic basis around the concept of gain. Strictly according to currently accepted criteria, gain from a cultural/societal perspective is not grounds for classifying that individual as having GID. Also excluded are intersex conditions such as genetic mosaicism, Klinefelter's syndrome and hormonal abnormalities such as congenital adrenal hyperplasia.

Diagnosis

Although there are diagnostic criteria as to what constitutes GID, it should be stated that the basic premise that it is a mental illness has been challenged. Some opinion sees parallels to the way that homosexuality was medicalized as an illness until recently, before it was removed from the DSM in the 1970s.

The best-known standards of care are from the Harry Benjamin International Gender Disorder Association (HBIGDA); the most up-to-date standards are version 6, revised in 2001 (HBSOC v6, 2001). The overarching goal of the Standards is to provide lasting personal comfort for the individual through a combination of medical, surgical and psychological interventions aimed at maximizing self-esteem, self-fulfilment and well-being. Diagnosis and management of this patient group is always multidisciplinary. Ideally, the team should include an endocrinologist or a physician with expertise in prescribing hormone therapy, a psychiatrist, a psychologist, the specialist surgeon and the patient's GP. Specialist voluntary sector organizations with an interest in the condition can provide exceptional peer support and counselling. The guidelines are not proscriptive, and recognize that a flexibility is required to tailor treatment options to the individual's needs.

Ethical considerations

The Harry Benjamin International Gender Dysphoria Association also publishes an ethical framework in which it expects practitioners to operate. There is an American slant to the published document, but much of what is stated is covered by the General Medical Council (GMC) documents on confidentiality and duty of care to patients. Guideline 9 is quoted in full:

> Members shall make decisions regarding care based solely on sound professional practices, without regard to race, religion, sexual orientation (including non-stereotypical or non-cultural gender role presentations), nationality, or age (unless related to medical conditions which preclude certain treatments). HIV status shall not be considered in the decision to evaluate or treat patients.

Although not explicit in the guidelines, a lower age of 18 is strongly recommended in the UK field of practice. Other countries, e.g. Holland and recently Australia, have begun medical treatment in pre-pubertal patients. Although this may sound contentious, it makes medical sense because of the complex and overwhelming changes that puberty produces, in these patients in an unwanted manner.

Legal framework within the UK

It is possible to change name by deed poll, obtain a new driving licence and new bank account under existing legislation. This would be expected during the real-life test (see below).

Recent changes to the laws of the United Kingdom, with particular reference to Human Rights legislation, have been very positive in trying to tackle deep-seated fears around stigmatization, employment and freedom to associate. Currently the Gender Recognition Bill is being debated in the House of Lords; this would allow a birth certificate to be changed to reflect the new gender. The implications of this legislation on inheritance are currently unclear.

Management of patients with gender dysphoria

Every patient is unique, often with complex psychological problems secondary to many years of gender conflict. Feelings of isolation, stigmatization and fear of rejection are common. A full, detailed and tactful history by an experienced member of the gender team, usually the psychiatrist, is a first stage. A history of the patient 'feeling trapped in the wrong body' from an early age is very common. Early childhood should also be explored, including relationships with parents, sibs, other family members and at school. It is important to explore the patient's sexual orientation, which is usually formed in the teenage years. While the patient's sexual orientation is useful in informing the overall picture and perhaps influencing the type of surgery, it is quite separate from the underlying diagnosis – a transsexual patient can be homosexual, bisexual or heterosexual.

Further aspects of history, including past history; family history, particularly of propensity to thrombotic episodes; and smoking history are also relevant. A clinical examination should include blood pressure, a check for varicose veins, (as a predisposing factor for venous thrombosis) and external genitalia if permitted. Many patients will refuse this last request unless absolutely necessary. Karyotyping studies are usually not indicated, but liver function tests, hormone profile (follicle stimulating hormone (FSH), luteinizing hormone (LH), testosterone/oestradiol, prolactin and sometimes adrenal hormones), haematology and bone density are usually performed. There may be a place for thrombophilia testing as per family or past medical history if oestrogen therapy is being contemplated.

Having identified a GID, triadic therapy should follow. In the usual sequence it would be:

- real-life test for 12 months (some authorities would say 24 months), see below
- hormone therapy, see below
- surgical change.

There is a logic to this sequence, although earlier use of hormones has been advocated. The irreversible nature of surgical treatment makes it important that the diagnosis is reviewed regularly, and the patient's views on this must be paramount. Some authorities insist on two independent reports on the patient's progress in the real-life test before surgery is undertaken.

Hormone therapy

With regards to hormonal therapy, the HBIGDA guidelines set three criteria. Firstly, patients should be over 18. Secondly, they should be aware of the effects and risks of taking the drugs. And thirdly, they should have documented proof that they were living in their desired gender role for at least 3 months (known as the 'real life experience'), or have undergone a minimum of 3 months of psychotherapy.

Cross-sex hormonal treatments play an important role in the anatomical and psychological gender transition process for properly selected adults with GIDs. Hormones are often medically necessary for successful living in the new gender. They improve the quality of life and limit psychiatric co-morbidity, which often accompanies lack of treatment. When physicians administer androgens to biologic females and oestrogens, progesterone, and testosterone-blocking agents to biologic males, patients feel and appear more like members of their preferred gender.

Male-to-female patients are treated with oestrogens. The safest preparation is oestradiol via the transdermal route, e.g. Estraderm MX 100-mg patches twice weekly. Bypassing the liver appears to reduce the risk of thromboembolism. Oral oestrogens, e.g. Premarin or Stilboestrol, are still occasionally used. The starting dose of Premarin for a patient is 1.25 mg, but doses of 7.5 mg per day are occasionally prescribed. Much of this is tailored to patient response to therapy, but the higher the dose, the more likely are side effects. Patients can expect to experience: breast growth and some redistribution of body fat in line with a more feminine appearance, decreased upper body strength, softening of the skin, a decrease in body hair, slowing or stopping of loss of scalp hair, decreased fertility and testicular size, and less frequent and less firm erections. These changes can take time to develop, and periods of up to 2 years may be required to see a full effect. Gynaecomastia is likely with treatment, but often the result is disappointing. Augmentation mammoplasty may then be indicated. Provera 5 mg b.d. for 3–6 months may help ductal breast tissue development.

Adjunctive treatments are usually undertaken too, e.g. speech therapy and electrolysis or other forms of depilation. Many authorities use cyproterone, finasteride or spironolactone as an anti-androgen preparation in male-to-female patients, and interval orchidectomy has also been reported prior to full gender surgery. Preservation of scrotal skin is necessary in this latter context.

Female-to-male patients are treated with testosterone. This can be as Sustanon injections, Andropatch or Testogel dermal preparations, or by a 400- to 600-mg implant subcutaneously every 4–6 months. Patients can expect the following permanent changes: a deepening of the voice, clitoral enlargement, reduction in breast size, more facial and body hair, and male pattern baldness. Reversible changes include increased upper body strength, weight gain, increased sex drive, and decreased hip fat.

Surgical therapy

A full discussion of the surgical procedures available is outwith the scope of this chapter. A reference is give for further reading for the interested individual.

With regard to surgery, there are six eligibility criteria within the Standards, the most important of which are that the patient should be a legal adult, have had 12 months of continuous hormone therapy and have lived in their desired gender role for a year. There are also two 'readiness' criteria. Patients should demonstrate that they are consolidating their gender identity and enjoy better mental health as a result of dealing effectively with work, their family and relationships. Psychiatrists are required to check that patients meet these criteria.

Male-to-female surgery
Once the necessary agreements have been met within the multidisciplinary team members, genital tract surgery is performed. The penis and testes are removed, the scrotal skin fashioning part of the neovagina. In variations of the procedure, part of the descending colon is used to fashion a neovagina, but this is a more complicated procedure. Preservation of the glans penis to construct a clitoris has also been described.

A simpler process of penile amputation and orchidectomy can be undertaken if there is no specific need to have a neovagina, e.g. if no penetrative sexual activity is planned. A test case in Sheffield a few years ago means that all health funding authorities should provide this as part of NHS care.

Other procedures, e.g. breast surgery and thyroid cartilage shaving can be undertaken; the list is extensive, but usually private funding is required.

Female-to-male surgery
This is performed in stages. Usually a mastectomy is performed first, followed by hysterectomy and oophorectomy. Construction of a phallus with the necessary urethral extension and erectile tissue is extremely specialized and is only performed in a few centres in the UK. For this reason, many patients elect to stop after the hysterectomy.

Further reading

Futterweit W. Endocrine therapy of transsexualism and potential complications of long-term treatment. Arch Sexual Behav 1998;27:209–26.

Harry Benjamin International Gender Dysphoria Association Standards of Care for Gender Identity Disorders version 6. www.hbigda.org

Mind. Understanding gender dysphoria (leaflet available directly from the charity).

Van Kesteren PJM, Asscheman H, Megens JAJ et al. Mortality and morbidity in transsexual subjects treated with cross-sex hormones. Clin Endocrinol 1997;47:337–42.

Appendix

International Classification of Diseases-10 (ICD-10)

ICD-10 now provides five diagnoses for gender identity disorders (F64):

Transsexualism (F64.0) has three criteria:
- The desire to live and be accepted as a member of the opposite sex, usually accompanied by the wish to make his or her body as congruent as possible with the preferred sex through surgery and hormone treatment;
- The transsexual identity has been present persistently for at least 2 years;
- The disorder is not a symptom of another mental disorder or a chromosomal abnormality.

Dual-role Transvestism (F64.1) has three criteria:
- The individual wears clothes of the opposite sex in order to experience temporary membership in the opposite sex;
- There is no sexual motivation for the cross-dressing;
- The individual has no desire for a permanent change to the opposite sex.

Gender Identity Disorder of Childhood (64.2) has separate criteria for girls and for boys.

For girls:
- The individual shows persistent and intense distress about being a girl, and has a stated desire to be a boy (not merely a desire for any perceived cultural advantages to being a boy) or insists that she is a boy;
- Either of the following must be present:
  - Persistent marked aversion to normative feminine clothing and insistence on wearing stereotypical masculine clothing;
  - Persistent repudiation of female anatomical structures, as evidenced by at least one of the following:
    An assertion that she has, or will grow, a penis;
    Rejection of urination in a sitting position;
    Assertion that she does not want to grow breasts or menstruate.
- The girl has not yet reached puberty;
- The disorder must have been present for at least 6 months.

For boys:
- The individual shows persistent and intense distress about being a boy, and has a desire to be a girl, or, more rarely, insists that he is a girl.
- Either of the following must be present:
  - Preoccupation with stereotypic female activities, as shown by a preference for either cross-dressing or simulating female attire, or by an intense desire to participate in the games and pastimes of girls and rejection of stereotypical male toys, games and activities;

- Persistent repudiation of male anatomical structures, as evidenced by at least one of the following repeated assertions:
  That he will grow up to become a woman (not merely in the role);
  That his penis or testes are disgusting or will disappear;
  That it would be better not to have a penis or testes.
- The boy has not yet reached puberty;
- The disorder must have been present for at least 6 months.

Other Gender Identity Disorders (F64.8) have no specific criteria.

Gender Identity Disorder, Unspecified has no specific criteria.

Either of the previous two diagnoses could be used for those with an intersex condition

Unwanted pregnancy and induced abortion

Gillian Flett

Induced abortion is one of the most commonly performed gynaecological procedures in Great Britain. Around 180 000 terminations are performed annually in England and Wales and around 12 000 in Scotland. Around 1 in 3 British women will have had an abortion by the age of 45. Over 98% of abortions in Britain are undertaken on the grounds that the pregnancy threatens the mental or physical health of the woman or her children. It is these abortions which form the focus of this review.

Access to NHS abortion provision varies considerably, with over 98% of terminations in Scotland being undertaken in NHS hospitals, in contrast with England and Wales where NHS agency arrangements complement NHS hospital provision and a significant proportion are obtained privately.

The law and abortion

Legal criteria for abortion are individual to the country of practice. It should be noted that in Northern Ireland, legal abortion is unavailable except to save the life of the mother or to prevent grave permanent injury to her physical or mental health.

Current abortion legislation in Great Britain is based on the 1967 Abortion Act as amended by the Human Fertilisation Embryology Act 1990. Abortion is legal in Great Britain if two doctors decide in good faith that a particular pregnancy is associated with factors that satisfy one or more of five grounds specified in the Regulations. Most abortions are undertaken on statutory grounds C or D, which state that the pregnancy has not exceeded its 24th week and if it continues would involve risk greater than if the pregnancy were terminated of injury to the physical or mental health of the woman or of the existing children of her family. There are further legal requirements in relation to Certification Notification of abortion procedures and a Certificate signed by two medical practitioners authorizing the abortion requires to be retained for a period of at least 3 years and the 'operating' practitioner must complete a notification form for each termination. This form is forwarded to the Chief Medical Officer (CMO) for the relevant UK country within 7 days. Doctors looking after women requesting abortion care should also apply principles of good practice as described in the GMC document *Duties of a Doctor*. There is a conscientious objection clause within the Abortion Act and the British Medical Association (BMA) have produced a helpful overview on the legal and ethical position. Practitioners with a conscientious objection should provide advice and perform the preparatory steps for arranging an abortion if the request meets the legal requirements; this will usually include referral to another doctor as appropriate. Doctors and nurses have the right to refuse to take part in an abortion, but not to refuse to take part in any emergency treatment.

In general, in addition to fulfilling legal statute, a clinician will wish to be certain that a woman has considered her options carefully and is sure of her decision for abortion and gives informed consent. Gestation is a major determinant of options available for terminating a pregnancy and a decision is usually reached by the woman in consultation with her medical carers and pregnancy counsellor. The method chosen has to be acceptable to the woman as well as being safe and effective. Full guidelines for good practice have been published by The Royal College of Obstetricians and Gynaecologists (RCOG).

Choosing the method of abortion

Choice is now an integral part of abortion care and information; coupled with sensitive counselling, it is essential to help the woman in selecting an abortion method that is right for her and to optimize the abortion experience. The factors that determine an individual woman's choice for medical or surgical abortion are complex, but in brief, the chief advantages of surgical methods are that they are simple and quick and associated with a low risk of complication or failure. Medical methods are often favoured because they appear more physiological, like a miscarriage, and avoid the need for uterine instrumentation; they also have low rates of complication and failure. Some women can feel a lack of control over a surgical procedure, whereas others prefer that they remain unaware and that the procedure is undertaken by their clinician.

The late 1980s and 1990s saw exciting new developments in medical methods for early abortion and improvement of the medical methods for mid-trimester abortion. It is these developments that have extended patient choice and diversified the provision of abortion services. In 1991 the anti-progestogen mifepristone was licensed for termination of pregnancy up to 9 weeks' gestation, and since then an extensive literature has built up to support the safety, efficacy and acceptability of the medical regimen for early first-trimester abortion. In 1995 the licence was extended to include pregnancies of over 13 weeks' gestation. At present, the medical regimen is not licensed for use in women with pregnancies over 9 and less than 13 weeks' gestation, and the majority of abortions at these gestations remains surgical. A randomized trial has compared medical and surgical termination at 10–13 weeks' gestation and shown the medical regimen to be an effective alternative to surgery with high acceptability, and some units offer medical termination at these gestations.

Clinical practice in three larger Scottish units indicates that more than half of eligible women opt for medical methods when given a choice at early gestations of up to 9 weeks, and Scottish abortion statistics reveal that over 50% of all terminations in Scotland are now performed medically. Interestingly, the introduction of medical termination has not affected abortion rates overall. The introduction of medical abortion has been slower in England and Wales and there is significant variation in its provision across Health Authorities. Patient surveys further confirm that women value being offered a choice of method appropriate to the gestation of their pregnancy.

RCOG guidelines recommend that conventional suction termination should be avoided for gestations of less than 7 weeks on the basis that for these very early gestations the procedure is three times more likely to fail to remove the gestation sac than those performed at between 7 and 12 weeks. Although medical termination is advocated for these very early gestations of less than 7 weeks, current research is evaluating manual vacuum aspiration (MVA) under local anaesthetic using strict protocols.

Selection of the medical or surgical method for later abortion, particularly beyond 15 weeks, is usually dependent on the availability of health care personnel who are trained and willing to participate in late dilatation and evacuation (D+E). It is certainly true that as gestational age increases, the safety of second-trimester surgical abortion depends highly on the operator's skill and experience and the current situation is that clinics and clinicians usually set their limits for operative care based on these considerations. Regrettably, there has been no formal comparison in clinical trials between second-trimester dilatation and evacuation and the modern methods of medical mid-trimester termination. It should be noted that hysterotomy, with its associated high morbidity and mortality, has virtually disappeared from practice (Figure 1).

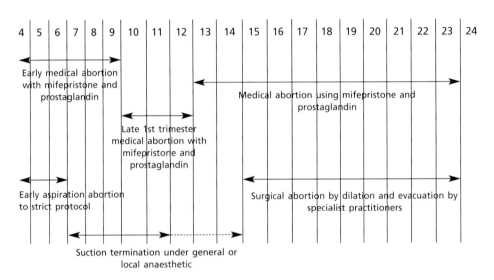

Figure 1 Methods of abortion at different gestations

Increasingly, women are referred to dedicated abortion services offering care separately from other gynaecological patients but with full gynaecological support should that be required. There is good supporting evidence that the earlier in pregnancy that an abortion is performed, the lower the risk of complications. Services should therefore be organized to offer arrangements which minimize delay for the patients. It is helpful if the referring doctor is able to provide the first signature on Certificate A. Day care is recognized as a cost-effective model of service provision and a typical service will be able to manage 90% of its patients on a day-care basis. Obviously, this will be influenced by pre-existing medical problems, social factors, geographical distance and the possibility of a planned day case requiring an overnight stay because of surgical or medical problems. Women undergoing mid-trimester termination, in particular, should be advised of the possible need for an overnight stay.

Pre-assessment for abortion

Counselling and procedure choice may well dominate the pre-assessment consultation, but it does provide an opportunity to screen for any pre-existing conditions that may require cross-specialty liaison and, despite the sensitivities of abortion, it is unusual for a woman to withhold her permission for such cross-consultation. It should be noted that for serious medical conditions, the risks of abortion are always lower than the risks of continued pregnancy. This visit also provides an opportunity for enquiry about previous use of contraception and discussion about intended use of contraception in an integrated manner.

Body mass index and blood pressure are checked at pre-assessment for all patients, and physical examination would be limited to auscultation of chest and heart for patients opting for general-anaesthetic surgical termination. An idea of gestational age will have been gained from the menstrual history, but given the inaccuracies of menstrual recall and limitations of bimanual pelvic examination, gestation is more accurately determined by ultrasound scan, either abdominal or vaginal, as relevant to the anticipated gestation. Viability and pregnancy location are also confirmed. This scan is undertaken in a sensitive setting and manner and the patient is advised that it is not necessary for her to watch the ultrasound examination in progress.

A full blood count can be useful to screen for anaemia and also acts as a baseline for comparison in the event of any substantial blood loss associated with the termination. This is also a useful opportunity to confirm immunity to rubella and to offer subsequent immunization if not immune. All patients have blood sent for confirmation of ABO and rhesus status with antibody screening. All unsensitized rhesus-negative women should be given anti-D immunoglobulin. Some centres offer testing for human immunodeficiency virus and hepatitis B and C at this time, but unless a policy for routine screening has been adopted and accepted, additional counselling would be required; in the meantime, such testing remains on a selective basis. Although not essential to abortion care, it is also an opportunity to check that cervical screening is up to date, and if it is not, opportunistic screening can be offered, ensuring that the result can be communicated to the women and appropriate action taken on any abnormal results.

Screening for genital tract infection helps to identify pathogens that increase the risk for post-abortion infection and pelvic inflammatory disease, as well as long-term sequelae of tubal infertility and ectopic pregnancy. The most important of these are *Chlamydia trachomatis* and *Neisseria gonorrhoeae*. A full screen, including for sexually transmitted infections (STI), allows for follow-up and partner notification and treatment to avoid re-infection. Some advocate antibiotic prophylaxis at the time of abortion, but prophylactic antibiotics alone do not allow for contact tracing and therefore leave women at risk from re-infection.

Some advocate the 'belt-and-braces' policy of a prophylactic regimen against chlamydia and bacterial vaginosis, along with a full STI screen. This is the approach in our own unit, where a prophylactic regimen of azithromycin 1 g orally and metronidazole 1 g rectally is offered to all women under 25 with a full screen offered to all women coming through the service.

Medical termination in the first trimester

The anti-progestogen mifepristone is used in combination with prostaglandin doses to achieve medical abortion. The contraindications to medical termination are few, but include suspected ectopic pregnancy, chronic adrenal failure, long-term steroid use, haemorrhagic disorders, treatment with anti-coagulants, known allergy to mifepristone or misoprostol, smokers over 35 years of age with electrocardiogram (ECG) abnormalities and breast-feeding women. Medical abortion is performed in hospital or premises registered for abortion. The patient attends briefly to take the mifepristone dose and attends subsequently for day-patient admission 36–48 hours later. It is customary for legal reasons to supervise the swallowing of the mifepristone tablets, but side effects are trivial and the women can leave after 10 minutes. Women may bleed slightly in the 48 hours after taking the mifepristone and a very small number may miscarry.

The prostaglandin route of administration and regimes vary and it is customary for the women to remain under supervision for 4–6 hours after prostaglandin administration, during which time the majority will expel the fetus. Nursing staff confirm passage of the products. The amount of bleeding is variable, often similar to a heavy period, and increases with gestation. A minority of women will have some lower abdominal cramp and will require oral analgesia and a minority (less than 5%) might require opiate analgesia. Length of gestation influences the success rate and complications, but this is more of an issue at 9–13 weeks' gestation. At these gestations, the risk of continuing pregnancy, in particular, remains a problem, and units undertaking medical termination at these gestations are cautious in counselling women regarding this. For women who pass minimal or no products of conception, ultrasound should be carried out. Unrecognized ongoing pregnancies would be of particular concern because of the risk of fetal abnormality.

Complete abortion rates of 97.5% are quoted for medical termination up to 9 weeks. At gestations over 9 and less than 13 weeks, in a review of 1076 medical terminations undertaken in Aberdeen, the complete abortion rate was 95.8%. The ongoing pregnancy rate was 1.5%. Surgical intervention is indicated for ongoing pregnancy, missed abortion, incomplete abortion and very heavy bleeding. The surgical intervention rate showed a progressive rise from 2.7% at 9–10 weeks' gestation to 8% at 12–13 weeks' gestation. All this is relevant to counselling the women about her choice, and of course is relevant to those involved in service planning. Data, however, is accumulating for the high uptake, acceptability and efficacy of medical termination at 9–13 weeks and, although still unlicensed at these gestations, it is likely to be offered as a choice for women undergoing abortion in many units.

Surgical termination

Surgical termination is performed in either a hospital or dedicated facility in a designated clinic. General anaesthesia is standard practice in the UK, although use of local anaesthesia (paracervical block) with or without sedation is increasingly being offered. Surgical termination is not recommended at less than 7 weeks' gestation because of the risk of failure to remove the pregnancy, but manual vacuum aspiration (MVA) is seeing renewed interest under strict protocols. For some women it is not appropriate to defer the abortion to a suitable gestation for surgery, and their preference might not be for medical abortion or indeed, in certain circumstances, there may be contraindications to medical abortion. For all surgical terminations there is evidence that cervical priming ahead of surgery reduces the complications of cervical injury, uterine perforation, haemorrhage and incomplete evacuation. The risk factors for cervical damage include younger patients and increasing gestation, especially in multiparous women. Gemeprost is the licensed preparation, although there is evidence from randomized controlled trials that misoprostol is an effective alternative that costs less and thus is frequently used.

Surgical termination is simple with low complication rates, but skill and experience are important so that serious complications are quickly recognized and remedied. Failed attempts at surgical abortion are recognized, with a quoted failure rate of 2.3 in 1000 abortions from a large series of women at less than 12 weeks' gestation. Sometimes this is explained by the presence of an unrecognized twin gestation or because the decidua will have been identified but the pregnancy not removed or there is a uterine anomaly. However, most failed surgical abortions occur in patients with normal pelvic anatomy and where the operator is experienced. It is prudent to advise patients regarding the possibility and to advise them to report any pregnancy symptoms persisting 1 week after the procedure so that evaluation for continuing pregnancy can take place and there can be early resort to further evacuation. Very rarely, even with full use of ultrasound, unusual situations can arise such as hetero-topic pregnancy (twin pregnancy with one embryo intra-uterine and one ectopic) and it is important to be mindful of such things when clinical history and findings are not straightforward. If there is any doubt about evacuation, the patient must be followed up.

Surgical abortion after the first trimester

Late dilatation and evacuation (D+E) is practised extensively in the US and there are skilled practitioners in England, the Netherlands, France and parts of Australia. It is not widely performed in other parts of the world. In Scotland, mid-trimester terminations are almost exclusively undertaken using modern medical methods. In England, D+E has not found favour among NHS gynaecologists but is more widely used by non-NHS abortion providers. Generally speaking, conventional first-trimester surgical evacuation can be used up to 15 weeks' gestation, but thereafter, specific techniques of cervical preparation and special instruments for D+E need to be used. Second-trimester abortion entails more risk than earlier procedures. More modern methods of aggressive cervical preparation coupled with extensive clinical experience of the procedure have improved safety. The use of ultrasound scanning during the procedure can also reduce perforation rates. This procedure can really only be safely undertaken by gynaecologists who have been specifically trained in the technique, have the specific instruments to perform the procedure and have a clinical through-put adequate for maintenance of skills. For some patients it could be a welcome choice, but D+E is not widely available and there is an absence of research evidence as to which technique is the safest and most appropriate for more advanced pregnancy.

Mid-trimester medical termination

Medical abortion is achieved at these gestations in a similar way to early medical termination by using oral mifepristone followed by repeated doses of prostaglandins 36–48 hours later. The regimes are safe and effective, although patients may experience minor side effects such as vomiting and diarrhoea associated with the procedure. The induction abortion interval tends to be longer with increasing gestation. Reported cumulative experience suggests that 97% of women abort successfully on the day of treatment within 5 doses of misoprostol. A second or third day of treatment may be required to complete the termination. Surgical evacuation under general anaesthetic may be required to complete the abortion and remove placental tissue. Published evidence suggests that this is required in about 8% of women and this fact should be incorporated into the counselling.

Complications and problems

Legal abortion in developed countries is impressively safe. Sadly, illegal, unsafe abortion remains a major contributor to maternal mortality on a global basis. The risk of complications is increased by older age, multiparity and increasing gestational age. Complications can be categorized into those that occur immediately at the time of the procedure and those that arise subsequently. Most of the immediate complications have been discussed in relation to the medical and surgical procedures outlined. The most common later complication is for a patient to present with problematic bleeding and/or pain where there may be retained products or infection. Ultrasound can be helpful in resolving the situation. Complex emotional feelings are often experienced immediately following termination and these include anger, guilt and regret and often contribute to short-term emotional distress. Most services offer follow-up counselling as required. The bulk of the evidence would support the view that abortion is very safe with few long-term problems, but patients do have concerns regarding their future reproductive health. There is no evidence to suggest that fertility difficulty or pregnancy complications are any more likely in patients who have had a previous abortion.

Conclusion

Legal induced abortion is one of the safest and commonest procedures in medicine. As with any other procedure, complications and failures are not completely avoidable, but they can be minimized by careful attention to detail by the medical providers using available published evidence and guidelines for practice. Gestation age should be accurately assessed and sound aseptic techniques used for interventionist procedures. Medical and nursing staff providing abortion services should be experienced and comfortable with the procedures and they must have a high index of suspicion for possible complications; the patient must have ready access to clinical services for post-abortion advice and the management of complications. The choice of abortion methods continues to extend with new developments and protocol refinements informed by ongoing research studies.

Further reading

Abortion statistics for Scotland, http://www.show.scot.nhs.uk/isd/index.htm

Ashok PW, Templeton A, Wagaarachchi PT, Flett GM. Factors affecting the outcome of early medical abortion: a review of 4132 consecutive cases. BJOG 2002;109(11):128–9.

Ashok PW, Templeton A, Wagaarachchi PT, Flett GM. Midtrimester medical termination of pregnancy: a review of 1002 consecutive cases. Contraception 2004;69(1):51–8.

Slade P, Hake S, Fletcher J, Stewart P. A comparison of medical and surgical termination of pregnancy: choice, emotional impact and satisfaction with care. Br J Obstet Gynaecol 1998; 105(12):1288–95.

Spitz IM, Bardin CW, Benton L, Robins A. Early pregnancy termination with mifepristone and misoprostol in the United States. N Engl J Med 1998;338(18):1241–7.

Westergaard L, Philipson T, Scheibel J. Significance of cervical *Chlamydia trachomatis* infection in post abortal pelvic inflammatory disease. Obstet Gynaecol 1982;60:322–5.

Urethral syndrome

Sunil Kumar and Raj Persad

Urethral syndrome is a condition seen commonly in women who present with dysuria and frequency suggestive of cystitis but the voided urine is sterile.

The syndrome consists of frequency, urgency, dysuria and suprapubic discomfort without any detectable abnormality to account for the symptoms. It is a diagnosis of exclusion and is sometimes difficult to distinguish from interstitial cystitis.

Causes

The precise aetiology is unknown, but the following possible causes have been suggested:

*   hormonal imbalance
*   reactions to environmental chemicals
*   allergies
*   psychological.

There is no robust evidence to support any of these possible causes.

Diagnosis

Urethral syndrome is a diagnosis of exclusion:

*   It is important to rule out infective causes (the presence of pyuria is a strong indicator of infection).
*   Atypical infections should be eliminated.
*   Gynaecological evaluation is often necessary as there is an important symptomatic overlap with gynaecological conditions in young women such as endometriosis or hormonal dysfunctions.
*   Urethrogram/MRI/transvaginal ultrasound scan may be performed to rule out urethral diverticulum.
*   Cystoscopy + hydrodistension +/– biopsies may be useful to rule out interstitial cystitis.
*   Urodynamics is of doubtful significance, but can sometimes unmask underlying atypical detrusor overactivity.

Management

- A course of antibiotics should be given even in the absence of positive cultures, especially if there is pyuria.
- Antibiotics should be selected to cover organisms such as chlamydia and anaerobes.
- Local oestrogen supplementation has been found to be effective in some cases.

Urethral dilatation is a procedure of historical interest only and there is no evidence base to suggest that the procedure has any benefit in this group of patients, although anecdotal reports abound.

Supportive treatment is essential as both the physician and the patient can find this condition extremely frustrating.

Vaginal discharge

Arnold Fernandes

Introduction

Women may present in a variety of settings (general practice, gynaecology, family planning or genitourinary medicine) with a complaint of vaginal discharge. There is no standard definition that differentiates a normal vaginal discharge from one that may be considered abnormal. However, an excessive or unpleasant vaginal secretion, with or without associated pruritus or genital odour, may be categorized as a working definition for an abnormal vaginal discharge.

Content of normal vaginal discharge

Physiological vaginal discharge is a conglomeration of secretions from various sources, including the vulva, Bartholin's glands, Skene's glands, vaginal transudate, cervical mucus and endometrial and tubal fluids. Cervical mucus is, however, the major component.

The amount and nature of the vaginal discharge varies with the age of the woman and the stage of her reproductive life, and in women of reproductive age, it varies with the phase of her menstrual cycle.

Vaginal secretions are normally acidic (pH 3.5–4.5) due to high lactic acid levels; the acid being formed by lactobacilli from the glycogen in vaginal epithelial cells. The acidity is maximal at birth and around the time of ovulation, and is minimal during childhood and post-menopausally.

Causes of vaginal discharge

- Physiological
  - pre-menstrually
  - around the time of ovulation
  - in the puerperium
  - post-abortal or post-termination of pregnancy.
- Associated with use of contraceptives
  - combined contraceptive pill
  - intrauterine contraceptive device.
- Non-infective microbial causes of discharge:
  - bacterial vaginosis (BV)
  - vaginal candidiasis.
- Sexually transmitted infections
  - *Neiserria gonorrhoeae*
  - *Chlamydia trachomatis*
  - *Trichomonas vaginalis* (TV).

- Less common infective causes of discharge
  - genital herpes
  - genital warts.
- Rare infective causes in the UK
  - syphilitic chancre
  - chancroid
  - granuloma inguinale.
- Associated gynaecological pathology
  - cervical lesions
  - cervical ectropion
  - cervical polyps
  - cervical neoplasia
  - trauma to the genital tract.
- Neoplasia of the genital tract
  - vagina
  - cervix
  - endometrium
  - fallopian tubes.
- Allergies to
  - soaps
  - deodorants
  - fabric conditioners.
- Retained foreign bodies in the genital tract
  - tampons (and toxic shock syndrome)
  - condoms.

Diagnosis

The following may be helpful in eliciting the cause of the discharge.

History

- Details of discharge: duration, consistency, odour, associated itchiness/soreness. For example, a smelly discharge could indicate BV or TV, an itch could suggest thrush or TV.
- Last menstrual period (LMP) and menstrual history including menstrual cycle, intermenstrual and post-coital bleeding. If bleeding is irregular, this could suggest chlamydia.
- Obstetric history, including recent miscarriage, delivery or termination of pregnancy.
- Abdominal/pelvic pain, dyspareunia, urinary symptoms.
- Previous cervical cytology.
- Past medical history: exclude diabetes, other immunosuppressive states.
- Sexual history.

Examination and diagnostic tests

- Thorough assessment of the external genitalia including inguinal nodes and vulva. For example, enlarged, tender inguinal nodes and a watery discharge could suggest herpes.
- Speculum examination to assess character of discharge.
- Assessment of vaginal pH. Useful if no access to on-site microscopy. pH above 4.5 would suggest BV or TV.
- High vaginal swab for microscopy and culture (lab will test for BV, yeast and TV).
- Cervical swab for gonorrhoea culture.
- Cervical swab for chlamydia test.
- Pelvic examination. May yield information in cases of upper-genital tract infections or associated gynaecological pathology.

Further Management

This depends on the cause. See the relevant sections for your suspected or confirmed diagnosis.

Physiological discharge can often be misconstrued as abnormal by women particularly if there has been a recent regretted sexual encounter; discussing this with the patient can often allay her anxieties.

Vulval pain

Susie Logan

Introduction

Vulvodynia is the medical term used to describe vulval pain. It is not a new condition, having been described over 100 years ago. It is a common symptom with many causes. While the majority of cases are not life-threatening, there can be life-ruining consequences, with women frequently suffering for many years. All too often it is assumed that the pain is caused by candidiasis. In general, vulval pain can be divided into four categories:

1. microbial (see page 79)
2. vulvar vestibulitis (see page 80)
3. dysaesthetic vulvodynia (see page 81)
4. others (see page 82)

The importance of a thorough history cannot be over-emphasized, as physical abnormalities are often absent. In addition to the vulva, examination should include the mouth and non-genital skin.

Symptoms

Depending on the cause, symptoms can include the following:

- stinging
- shooting pains
- hypersensitivity – hyperpathia
- allodynia – e.g. feeling a light touch as if it was burning
- rubbing
- cracking/splitting
- tenderness
- dryness
- burning/heat
- swelling
- painful walking
- painful sitting
- painful sex.

Causes

Microbial

Microbial causes of vulval pain include candidiasis, trichomoniasis and herpes simplex. See the relevant section of the book for information about these conditions.

Vulvar vestibulitis

The aetiology of this condition is unknown. Women often report that the symptoms follow a specific event, e.g. a severe attack of thrush. There is an association with interstitial cystitis, fibromyalgia and irritable bowel syndrome. Subsequent psycho-sexual problems are common.

Assessment

Women presenting with vulvar vestibulitis are usually Caucasian and under 40 years of age. They typically describe severe pain and discomfort of the vestibule (the region where the vulva meets with the vagina, including the Bartholin's and vestibular glands and the urethra). Pain is experienced when pressure is applied to the vestibule during sexual intercourse or insertion of tampons. The pain often continues for a variable period (hours to days) after sex. For some, even tight clothes or a light touch can cause symptoms. Itching is not usually present.

On examination, there is focal tenderness of the vestibule, usually worst near the Bartholin's ducts and Skene's glands (near the urethral meatus). There may be red areas (erythema) at the sites of tenderness, but often there are no signs of inflammation.

Diagnosis is made on clinical grounds, especially if vulval pain, focal tenderness and erythema are present. However, infections, particularly of *Candida*, should be screened for and a biopsy may be warranted to exclude other skin conditions.

Management

Spontaneous remission can occur in up to 50% of patients. General advice on vulval care (see appendix to this section) should be followed. Non-prescribed creams, e.g. over-the-counter thrush therapy, can cause vulval irritation and are best avoided. The treatment approach should address both the pathophysiological and psychological components of the condition, but treatment approaches lack the backing of well-designed trials.

Treatment options include:

1. Medication
   - Soothing agents – aqueous cream, emulsifying ointment, Emulsiderm bath lotion.
   - Topical local anaesthetic preparations – either applied half-an-hour prior to sexual intercourse or regularly.
   - Pain modifiers – amitriptyline/nortriptyline or gabapentin. The starting dose of amitriptyline is 10 mg nocte. The dose should be increased by 10 mg every 2 weeks, titrated against the response, to a maximum of 50 mg nocte. However, while amitriptyline is often used, there is no randomized-trial evidence to support this. Gabapentin can be used if the woman is intolerant to the side effects of tricyclics.
   - Topical steroids – alone and in combination with other agents, e.g. trimo-vate, if there is a coexisting inflammatory dermatosis, eg. eczema.
   - Oestrogen cream.

2. Therapy
   - Psychosexual counselling.
   - Behavioural therapy to train the introital muscles to relax:
     - vaginal trainers are graded in size
     - electromyographic biofeedback from a vaginal probe
     - perineal massage.
   - Pelvic floor muscle physiotherapy.

3. Surgery
   - The most common surgical procedure is a vestibulectomy. The amount of tissue removed is variable, depending on symptoms. Post-operative management may include the use of creams (steroid creams, emollients), vaginal trainers, or review by a pain management team or psychosexual counsellor. Reported success rates are extremely variable, ranging from 20% to over 90%. Surgery is effective only in well-selected patients and should be reserved for when non-invasive treatments fail. Complications include scar tissue formation, granulation tissue formation and infection.

Dysaesthetic vulvodynia

Dysaesthesia means altered sensation. This can include hyperpathia (where an otherwise mildly unpleasant stimulus can be agonizing) and allodynia (where a different sensation is felt from the one usually experienced, e.g. pressure may be perceived as burning). Again, the aetiology of dysaesthetic vulvodynia is unknown. It is hypothesized that vulval nerve fibres get irritated or damaged and fire abnormal nerve signals back to the spinal cord, resulting in pain. A similar clinical picture is seen in post-herpetic neuralgia.

Assessment

Women tend to be Caucasian, peri- or post-menopausal, and complain of long-standing vulval burning and soreness. The pain can vary from mild discomfort to severe pain that prevents comfortable sitting or sleeping. The pain may also affect the inside of the thighs, the upper legs, anus and urethra, Foreplay and penetration may also be painful. Itching is rarely a feature. Examination is often unremarkable, but it is helpful to delineate the affected area since this can clarify which nerve is affected.

Diagnosis is made on clinical grounds. Remember, however, that a minority will have referred vulval pain secondary to back problems causing spinal nerve compression, bladder and bowel pathology, and rectovaginal endometriosis.

Management

As with vulval vestibulitis, treatment options lack the backing of well-designed trials. Options include:

- vaginal lubricants – Sensilube, Astroglide
- soothing agents – aqueous cream, emulsifying ointment, Emulsiderm bath lotion
- topical local anaesthetic preparations – either applied half-an-hour prior to sexual intercourse or regularly

- pain modifiers – amitriptyline (up to 50 mg nocte), nortriptyline, carbamazepine, gabapentin or dothiepin
- complementary medication – aloe vera gel, Calendula, Dr Bach Rescue Cream, hypercal creams, Aveeno (see Appendix)
- complementary treatments – acupuncture and chiropractic
- Others – a combination of a low-oxalate diet and the drug calcium citrate (which removes oxalate from the body) is widely used in America, but less so in the UK. As the pain is more continuous, surgery is usually unsuccessful.

Other causes of vulval pain

These include, vulval intra-epithelial neoplasia, dermatitis, lichen sclerosus and lichen planus. See the relevant chapter for more information.

Pregnancy and vulval pain

Women who are pregnant are more prone to thrush infections. Some studies have suggested that among women with vulval vestibulitis, one-fifth noticed that their pain started following delivery. It is not clear whether this is a result of true vulval vestibulitis or pain from stitches, oestrogen deficiency while breast feeding or due to vaginal infections.

Sex and vulval pain

Sex that produces hymenal or posterior fourchette fissures can mimic vulval vestibulitis. The fissures can usually be seen if the woman is examined within 48 hours of intercourse.

Vulval pain impacts on sexual functioning, affecting both quality and frequency. Fear of pain or anticipation of pain during sex can result in vaginismus (involuntary spasm of the pelvic floor muscles surrounding the vagina, making penetration impossible), decreased libido and arousability, problems with orgasm and aversion to sex. Relationship difficulties inevitably result. Treatment approaches include biofeedback and behavioural and psychosexual therapy. Research suggests that these non-invasive approaches should be used before contemplating surgery. Sexual therapy is available privately and on the NHS. A list of accredited and registered sexual and relationship therapists is available from BASRT (British Association of Sexual and Relationship Therapy) and the IPM (Institute of Psychosexual Medicine). Relate (formerly Marriage Guidance) counsellors may also provide psychosexual therapy. Finally, qualified clinical psychologists may provide a service addressing both pain and sexual/relationship difficulties.

Conclusion

Women with vulval pain frequently suffer for many years. Early diagnosis in primary care with appropriate treatment and, if required, referral to a specialist vulval clinic, will expedite appropriate management. Supportive therapy in the form of explanation and reassurance is essential. Recent collaboration between gynaecologists, dermatologists, genitourinary medicine physicians, psychologists and psychosexual counsellors means that both physical and psychological aspects can now be addressed. However, specialists need to urgently direct their attention to proper evaluation of the plethora of unproven treatment options available and in use.

Further reading

BASRT (British Association of Sexual and Relationship Therapy), www.basmt.org.uk/
British Society for the Study of Vulval Diseases, www.bssvd.fsnet.co.uk
IPM (Institute of Psychosexual Medicine), www.ipm.org.uk
Skin Care Campaign, www.skincarecampaign.org
The Clinical Effectiveness Group (British Association of Sexual Health and HIV). National guidelines (2002) on the management of vulval conditions, vulvovaginal candidiasis, *Trichomonas vaginalis*, and genital herpes, www.bashh.org/ceguidelines.htm
The Vulval Pain Society is a volunteer UK organization that provides women with information about their condition. Their website (www.vul-pain.dircon.co.uk) has sections on different types of vulval pain; self-help suggestions; advice on pregnancy, contraception, surgery, diet and natural products; support groups; medical specialists by area; and links to other helpful sites.

Appendix

The following advice is adapted from the Vulval Pain Society's website (www.vulpain.dircon.co.uk/).

Self-help measures for vulval pain:

- Avoid soaps, bubble baths, deodorants or vaginal wipes, and coloured toilet paper in or around the vulval area. Clean the vulval area with water only, or with a soap substitute (aqueous cream BP or emulsifying ointment), preferably using showers not baths. Avoid antiseptics in the bath.
- When washing your hair, avoid allowing the shampoo from coming into contact with the vulval area.
- Clean the vulval area only once a day, avoiding scrubbing with flannels and brushes.
- Avoid overuse of creams that have not been prescribed.
- Wear loose-fitting, undyed cotton underwear and avoid tight-fitting garments.
- Try washing undergarments with water only. Fabric conditioners and washing powders contain potential irritants.
- Use unscented, unbleached tampons, sanitary towels/pads and panty liners, such as Natracare products (http://www.natra.dircon.co.uk/).
- Bathe the affected area in lukewarm, plain water (steeped tea water is an alternative). Add instant oatmeal, colloidal oatmeal (Aveeno), or baking soda.
- Use for 5–10 minutes two or more times a day, compresses of Aveeno (dissolved in water and stored in the fridge) or wet tea bags.
- If passing urine makes symptoms worse, wash the urine away from the vulval area using a jug of warm water while on the toilet. Use vitamin E oil several times a day, especially after urination.
- If swimming or exercising, protect the vulval area with Epiderm barrier cream. Avoid jacuzzis.
- If sex is painful, try using Biorex 5% lignocaine ointment just before intercourse (available from pharmacies without a prescription).
- Some women find that strengthening their pelvic-floor muscles using pelvic-floor or Kegel exercises can help reduce their symptoms (www.kegel-exercises.com).

Many condoms are scented and contain the spermicide nonoxynol-9 that can aggravate symptoms. Low-allergy condoms are available. Diaphragms and caps usually are used with a spermicidal cream, but some are available which use more natural products (e.g. honey) and are less irritating.

PART III

CONDITIONS

Bacterial vaginosis

Arnold Fernandes

Introduction

Bacterial vaginosis (BV) is the commonest cause of abnormal discharge in women of childbearing age. It is characterized by an overgrowth of predominantly anaerobic organisms. It can arise and remit spontaneously. It is not regarded as a sexually transmitted infection.

Presentation

Bacterial vaginosis is commonly diagnosed clinically by the presence of an offensive, non-irritant vaginal discharge. This is classically described as being thin, white or grey and homogenous and may coat the walls of the vagina and vestibule. The pH of the vaginal discharge is normally in the relatively alkaline range (>4.5)

It is important to remember that approximately 50% of women are asymptomatic.

Complications

- BV at the time of a termination of pregnancy has been associated with the development of post-termination of pregnancy (TOP) endometritis and upper genital tract infection.
- BV at the time of vaginal hysterectomy has been associated with an increased incidence of cuff cellulitis following hysterectomy.
- BV is associated with late miscarriage, pre-term birth, pre-term premature rupture of membranes and post-partum endometritis in pregnancy.

Diagnosis

Historically, BV was diagnosed by using Amsel's clinical criteria.

Amsel's criteria – at least three of the four criteria listed below needed to be present for the diagnosis to be confirmed:

- thin, white, homogenous, vaginal discharge
- clue cells on microscopy (these are epithelial cells covered with mixed organisms)
- pH of vaginal fluid > 4.5
- release of a fishy odour on adding alkali (10% KOH) to a specimen of the vaginal discharge.

Diagnosis by microscopy

In more recent years, microscopy of a Gram-stained vaginal smear has become a popular method of diagnosis. The techniques vary from detailed counting of different morphological bacterial types (Nugent criteria) to categorizing the flora into grades (Hay–Ison criteria).

In clinical situations, the grading system described by Hay et al is commonly used to make the diagnosis. The grading system is shown below:

- **Grade 0** – epithelial cells only with no bacteria.
- **Grade 1** – normal vaginal flora (lactobacillus morphotypes only – this is a normal smear).
- **Grade 2** – intermediate vaginal flora, i.e. reduced number of lactobacillus morphotypes with a mixed bacterial flora. This grade is believed to be a transitional phase between the normal and BV state.
- **Grade 3** – few or no lactobacilli (indicative of BV). Many different bacteria, both Gram-positive and Gram-negative are seen, which give a 'salt and pepper' appearance. 'Clue cells' are present in the majority of these smears but it is the appearance of the mixed flora that is indicative of BV.
- **Grade 4** – other pattern, e.g. just streptococci with no lactobacilli or organisms associated with BV. Sometimes seen in smears from post-menopausal women.

Isolation of *Gardnerella vaginalis* cannot be used to diagnose BV.

Treatment

Treatment is only indicated for symptomatic women, some pregnant women (see below) or those undergoing gynaecological surgery.

First-line treatment for bacterial vaginosis involves the use of metronidazole in a dose of 400 mg twice daily for 5 days. Alternatively, 2 g of metronidazole may be used as a single oral dose. Metronidazole needs to be taken on a full stomach. Alcohol should be avoided because of an Antabuse-like reaction that may develop.

Alternative regimens include intravaginal metronidazole gel (0.75%) used once daily for 5 days, **or** intravaginal clindamycin cream (2%) used once daily for 7 days **or** clindamycin (300 mg) taken orally twice daily for 7 days.

Oral clindamycin can cause pseudo-membranous colitis and clindamycin cream can weaken condoms.

Metronidazole allergy is uncommon. Clindamycin cream 2% is recommended for women who are allergic to metronidazole.

Recurrent bacterial vaginosis

There are few published studies evaluating the optimal approach to treating this group of women. Small studies using Aci-jel, live yoghurt or *Lactobacillus acidophilus* have not demonstrated a benefit. One anecdotal suggestion is to try a standard 5-day course of metronidazole 400 mg b.d. followed by suppression with weekly vaginal metronidazole gel or clindamycin cream for a few months.

Women with recurrent BV are advised to avoid vaginal douching and the use of shower gel, antiseptic agents or shampoo in the bath.

Pregnancy and breast feeding

A number of randomized controlled trials have shown that women with a history of prior idiopathic pre-term birth or second trimester loss should be screened for BV and receive treatment with a course of oral metronidazole, preferably early in the second trimester of pregnancy.

The results of further randomized controlled trials of screening and treating all pregnant women are awaited. One recently published study highlighted that treatment of pregnant women with asymptomatic abnormal vaginal flora and BV with oral clindamycin early in the second trimester significantly reduced the rate of late miscarriage and spontaneous pre-term birth in a general obstetric population.

Although, meta-analyses have concluded that there is no evidence of teratogenicity from the use of metronidazole in women during the first trimester of pregnancy, it is best to avoid use of metronidazole in the first trimester. Clindamycin 300 mg twice daily for 7 days can be used if metronidazole is contraindicated.

It is prudent to use an intravaginal treatment for lactating women because oral metronidazole can make breast milk unpalatable.

Following treatment for bacterial vaginosis, a test of cure is not necessary. If, however, treatment is prescribed in pregnancy to reduce the risks of pre-term birth, a repeat test should be performed after 1 month and further treatment offered if the BV has recurred.

Management of sexual partners

Screening and treatment of sexual partners is not indicated as the current view is that BV is not transmitted sexually.

Other management

Any woman presenting with vaginal discharge should have a sexual history taken and be advised to have a screen for STIs.

Further reading

Hay P. National guideline for the management of bacterial vaginosis.
  http://www.bashh.org/guidelines/ceguidelines.htm

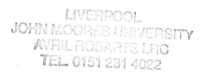

Chancroid

Steve Baguley

Introduction

Chancroid is an ulcerating infection caused by *Haemophilus ducreyi*, a Gram-negative coccobacillus. Until the middle of the 20th century, the condition was endemic in most parts of the world. Indeed it was one of the original venereal diseases named in the English and Welsh VD Act of 1916 (along with gonorrhoea and syphilis).

Cases have declined significantly since then – this is thought to be partially due to changes in the sex industry. Compared to 1900 there are now more job opportunities for poor urban women and for those who do enter the sex industry there has been an improvement in their working lives and health. Chancroid relies on frequent partner change to spread in a community and because its symptoms are painful, when medical attention is available, people seek help rather than have more sex.

It is now very rare in the UK, with only a few dozen cases diagnosed in UK GUM clinics in 2002. In the same year, 69 cases were reported in the US. In post-industrial nations, most cases occur in people with a history of sexual contact with someone from a country where chancroid is more common. Sporadic outbreaks do occur, however, and tend to be in groups where sex is exchanged for drugs. Such outbreaks are usually rapidly brought under control by thorough partner notification. Chancroid is still endemic in many countries of South and West Africa and in parts of South East Asia. For example, in 2000 a study in Botswana found that 26% of genital ulcers were caused by *H. ducreyi*.

Because of the popularity of international travel and the increasing role of crack cocaine in the European sex industry, there is still a chance of coming across the condition.

Presentation

Unlike many STIs the majority of people with chancroid have symptoms, although some women can be asymptomatic.

Chancroid is most likely to present as genital ulceration. Two to ten days after acquisition a papule appears. This then ruptures leaving an ulcer. Most people have more than one lesion and they are typically deeper than herpetic ulcers with an irregular edge and a sloughy base. They are soft and painful, which distinguishes them from the chancres of primary syphilis. Size varies from a few millimetres to several centimetres. Co-infection with herpes simplex virus or *Treponema pallidum pallidum* can alter the appearance. In people with HIV, the ulcers can be unusually persistent and more likely to be extragenital.

Cervical lesions can present with dyspareunia; vulval lesions can cause dysuria; and rectal lesions can cause rectal pain or bleeding. Unlike in herpes, a flu-like prodrome does not occur.

Auto-inoculation to other sites such as the thighs and hands can occur.

One or two weeks following the appearance of the ulcers, most people develop regional lymphadenitis. This is usually inguinal, unilateral and painful. The lymph node can necrose and ulcerate through the skin.

Complications

Ulcers can lead to tissue destruction and bleeding if they erode into blood vessels. Secondary infection can delay healing and contribute to tissue damage. Sometimes fistulae form which are slow to heal. The lesions usually heal with scarring and this can result in phimosis or anal stenosis.

Haematogenous or lymphatic dissemination to distant sites does not occur.

Chancroid is a cofactor for the transmission of HIV.

Diagnosis

The diagnosis should be suspected in anyone with typical symptoms who has had sex with someone from a country where chancroid is common. There are very few other causes of tender, fluctuant inguinal node enlargement. It is essential to try to confirm the diagnosis, however, due to the implications for partner notification.

H. ducreyi can be grown but this needs specialized transport and culture media which are not widely available.

Gram-stained microscopy of material taken from an ulcer or bubo can identify the Gram-negative coccobacilli that often cluster in a 'school of fish' pattern.

Unfortunately, due to the numerous other organisms seen in genital ulcers, microscopy has low sensitivity and specificity.

PCR tests are becoming more widely available and are the most sensitive method – check with your local lab whether they can provide this service.

Treatment

Azithromycin 1 g p.o. once is very effective, although follow-up is essential since treatment failures can occur. Resistance to azithromycin is currently very unusual but will undoubtedly become more common as its use increases.

Buboes can be aspirated or incised and drained under antibiotic cover.

Other management

The patient should be offered a check for other STIs, including other causes of genital ulceration, and HIV. The patient should be followed up at about 5 days and again if the ulcers have not healed. If the ulcers have not healed, it might be because they were very large, the person could have HIV, the *H. ducreyi* might be resistant to azithromycin or it might not be chancroid.

Give advice about reducing risk of acquiring STIs in the future.

Sexual contacts

All sexual contacts since 2 weeks prior to onset of ulceration should be seen and examined. The person should be advised to avoid sex until the lesions have completely healed.

Further reading

Mayaud P, McCormick D. UK national guidelines on the management of chancroid. 2001. http://www.bashh.org/guidelines/chancroid%2009%2001b.pdf

Chlamydia trachomatis

Steve Baguley

Introduction and epidemiology

Chlamydia trachomatis causes several diseases including trachoma (scarring conjunctivitis and a common cause of blindness – not covered in this book) and lymphogranuloma venereum (see page 141). However most people associate the organism with genital chlamydia infection or just plain 'chlamydia', and this final disease is what will be covered in this section.

The different subtypes of *C. trachomatis* are characterized by the immune response to one of the membrane proteins. By this process, serovars A to L3 can be identified; genital chlamydia infection is caused by types D to K. The significance of knowing which serovar is causing someone's pelvic inflammatory disease or urethral discharge is currently unclear, although some serovars do appear to be associated with more severe symptoms. Because of the uncertain clinical relevance, serotyping or genotyping is currently only done in a research setting.

Diagnoses of chlamydia have increased significantly since the mid-1990s. This is due to a number of factors, including better diagnostic tests and more people being tested. Because chlamydia generally causes no symptoms, many diagnoses are made as a result of people being offered a test when they were attending their GP, for example, for an unrelated reason. It is therefore unclear what is happening to the true incidence or prevalence of chlamydia. What is clear though is that chlamydia is very common. Prevalence estimates vary widely depending on the age group and population studied. Figures from the UK suggest that 10–15% of sexually active teenagers have the infection, although rates in the 40-plus age group are probably less than 3%. The highest prevalence rates are generally found in sexually active teenage women. The high rates in young people are thought to be due to relatively frequent partner changes in this age group and possibly due to the use of the combined oral contraceptive, which makes women more susceptible to the infection. Another hypothesis is that it might have something to do with immunity – a woman in her 40s who has already had chlamydia twice might be better able to spontaneously clear the infection.

Chlamydia can be transmitted by vaginal, anal and oral sex (fellatio). It can probably also be transmitted by non-penetrative genital contact – for example the penile tip touching the vulval vestibule.

Presentation

Chlamydia is well known for only rarely causing symptoms. Its ability to exist in a latent state within the columnar epithelium of the cervix and urethra means that it usually causes little inflammatory reaction. It can exist in this way for a considerable period, perhaps only being detected years into a monogamous relationship, prompting unfounded accusations of infidelity.

Perhaps the commonest presentation for chlamydia is therefore an asymptomatic person who wanted a check up or who was a contact of someone with the infection. However, about 10% of women and 20% of infected men do have symptoms.

For men these include:

- dysuria – discomfort when passing urine
- urethral discharge – often very slight or clear
- painful testes or epididymitis (suggests possible epididymo-orchitis – see page 99).

Some men who claim to be symptom free turn out to have a noticeable discharge when examined.

Women with symptoms might complain of:

- an abnormal vaginal discharge – heavy or green/yellow tinged
- bleeding between periods or after sex
- dysuria
- pelvic pain
- deep dyspareunia – pelvic pain during sex (pelvic pain suggests possible pelvic inflammatory disease, see page 152).

Rectal and pharyngeal infections are almost always asymptomatic. If you diagnose someone with rectal chlamydia who has symptoms of proctitis or urethral chlamydia with inguinal lymphadenopathy, consider lymphogranuloma venereum (see page 141).

Complications

Numerous magazine articles have concentrated on the risk of infertility that chlamydia brings. It is hard to estimate exactly how likely this is since it would require a large 'natural history' study, and that would be unethical. However, it appears to be an uncommon late complication with perhaps a few percent of infected women at most developing tubal factor infertility and/or ectopic pregnancies. Despite being a rare outcome, this has a huge impact on public health because chlamydia is so common. (See Pelvic inflammatory disease, page 152, for more information). It is debatable whether chlamydia has any effect on male fertility.

Apart from infertility, chlamydia can cause numerous other complications including:

In men
- epididymo-orchitis (see page 99).

In women
- miscarriage, stillbirth and other complications
- pelvic inflammatory disease (see page 152).

In men and women
- Reiter's syndrome/sexually acquired reactive arthritis (and rarely pneumonitis, meningoencephalitis, endocarditis) see page 165
- conjunctivitis.

In neonates
- pneumonitis
- conjunctivitis.

Diagnosis

Several diagnostic tests for chlamydia exist, including culture, immunofluorescence microscopy, enzyme immunoassays (EIAs) and nucleic acid amplification tests (NAATS). NAATS generally offer the best performance in that they are quite sensitive (85–95%) and specific (90–98%); analysis can be automated and specimens can include self-collected material such as urine. However, they are more expensive than EIAs, which is why they have not been universally adopted.

It is important to know which test your laboratory uses because it will alter the specimen collection methods that are available. It will also alter interpretation of the results; is this negative result really negative, or could it be a false negative?

Assuming that your laboratory can carry out NAATs, appropriate specimens for a man are either a first-void urine specimen (first 20 ml of urine voided having held urine for a minimum of an hour) or a urethral swab. Special swabs are usually needed – check with the lab.

For a woman, appropriate specimens are first-void urine, an endocervical swab and a self-obtained low vaginal swab.

NAATs and EIAs are unlicensed for use on specimens obtained from the rectum and pharynx, although NAATs are increasingly being used on specimens obtained from these sites. Validation studies will be required to ensure that these results are being interpreted correctly.

Treatment

For management of pelvic inflammatory disease see page 155. For management of epididymo-orchitis see page 100.

For uncomplicated infections, including pharyngeal, rectal and conjunctival infections, use azithromycin 1 g p.o. once (good adherence, relatively expensive, cure rate >95%) or, if not pregnant, doxycycline 100 mg p.o. b.d. for 7 days (cheaper, cure rate >95%).

Pregnancy and breast feeding

If the patient is pregnant, the UK guidelines recommend using erythromycin 500 mg twice daily for 2 weeks. However, azithromycin is better tolerated in pregnancy and appears to be safe. It is also more effective.

Patients should avoid sexual contact for a week after starting azithromycin or doxycycline; if using erythromycin, they should avoid sex until they have had a negative test of cure at 3 weeks.

Sexual contacts

About 70% of sexual contacts will have chlamydia themselves, so all recent contacts need to be seen, tested and in most cases given 'epidemiological' treatment before results are available. Partners should be given treatment at this stage for two reasons – they may have sex before they are seen again or the test may be falsely negative and so they may unwittingly spread the infection to others. See page 10 for advice on partner notification.

Other management

If the person has so far just had a test for chlamydia, they should be offered a test for other STIs including gonorrhoea, syphilis and HIV.

In most cases the person will have caught the infection by having sex without a condom. Therefore they need to be given advice about having safer sex in the future. They should be given written information about the infection and possible complications.

Follow up

People may need to be seen again or phoned to discuss progress with partner notification. It used to be recommended that people should have a test of cure (TOC). However, with the use of effective antibiotics such as azithromycin and doxycycline, this is no longer necessary unless symptoms persist. A test of cure should, however, be done if alternative agents are used such as erythromycin. Because most tests for chlamydia pick up non-viable organisms, this should be done a minimum of 3 weeks after treatment to allow for clearance.

Although a TOC is of limited value, a test of reinfection can be useful since a significant minority of people will have a positive test if re-examined several months following treatment. Some UK GUM clinics are therefore advising a repeat test at 3–6 months.

Further reading

http://www.chlamydiae.com/ everything you ever wanted to know about *C. trachomatis* and other chlamydia species.

Management of genital *Chlamydia trachomatis* infection. Scottish intercollegiate guideline network. http://www.sign.ac.uk/guidelines/fulltext/42/.

Donovanosis

Steve Baguley

Introduction

Donovanosis is caused by *Klebsiella granulomatis*, a Gram-negative bacillus with a variable appearance. Most cases occur in the Caribbean and South East Asia. Cases are also reported from Northern Australia, although diagnoses have declined since the government launched an eradication program. Donovanosis is rare in the UK with only a few dozen cases reported each year. However, the relentless rise in international travel and condom-free sex will mean that some readers will come across the occasional case.

Presentation

The classic lesion is a denuded area of skin with a clean, friable, dark-red surface. Although initially covering only a small area, the lesions can progressively enlarge to be well over 10 cm in diameter. Although classed as an ulcerating disease, the granulating lesions of Donovanosis can initially be papular. Larger ulcers can be very smelly. Genital skin is the most likely area to be affected, but other sites can be involved, including subcutaneous tissues as well as deeper structures such as pelvic organs and bone.

When subcutaneous tissue in the groin is affected, it can give the impression of lymphadenopathy, so the term pseudobubo is used. Lesions of the cervix and uterus are usually clinically diagnosed as neoplasms. Bone lesions are often taken to be due to tuberculosis.

The diagnosis should be considered in anyone presenting with these symptoms who gives a history of sex with a national of a country where the infection is endemic.

Complications

- Genital lesions can lead to massive tissue destruction including penile amputation.
- Lymphatic destruction can result in lymphoedema. Vertebral involvement can lead to spinal compression.
- Vertical transmission can occur.
- A small proportion of cases progress to squamous cell carcinoma.

Diagnosis

In view of the differential diagnosis, clinical suspicion should always be confirmed. The best way is by microscopy of a piece of crushed granulation tissue. The tissue can be obtained by scraping the base of an ulcer with a tongue depressor (the lesions are usually only mildly tender) or by a pinch or punch biopsy. The garnered material is then crushed between a couple of slides and air dried. Warthin–Starry or Wright–Giemsa stains are used to demonstrate *K. granulomatis* within macrophages. The typical appearance is of a closed safety pin. Immature forms exist within intracytoplasmic vacuoles called Donovan bodies.

PCR tests are available, although not widely.

Treatment

K. granulomatis is sensitive to numerous antibiotics, but in Australia, azithromycin has been found to be very effective. It is usually given at a dose of 1 g per week until lesions have completely healed. Lesions can recur up to 18 months after resolution.

Other management

The person should be offered a check for other STIs including HIV. Other management will depend on the sites affected.

Sexual contacts

All sexual contacts since 2 months prior to onset of ulceration should be seen and examined. The person should be advised to avoid sex until the lesions have completely healed.

Further reading

Richens J. UK guideline on the management of Donovanosis. 2001. http://www.bashh.org/guidelines/donovanosis%2009%2001b.pdf

Epididymitis

Sunil Kumar and Raj Persad

The epididymis is the convoluted tube from the testis that becomes the vas deferens; it is important for the transport and maturation of sperm from the testis. Infection of the epididymis is not uncommon in elderly men with bladder outflow obstruction and lower urinary tract infection (usually due to prostatic enlargement) but it can also occur in younger and sexually active males. The predominant organisms vary according to age.

Acute epididymitis is characterized by severe testicular pain and swelling of less than 6 weeks duration.

Causes

Infective causes include:

- sexually acquired
  - *Chlamydia trachomatis* (commonest) (≤ 35 yrs of age)
  - *Neisseria gonorrhoea*
- bacterial infection
  - *Escherichia coli* (in men practising unprotected anal intercourse)
  - *Proteus*
  - *Klebsiella*
  - *Pseudomonas.*
- other infection
  - *Mycobacterium tuberculosis*
  - *Candida albicans*
  - mumps

Non-infective causes include:

- amiodarone therapy
- polyarteritis nodosa (PAN)
- vasculitis
- Henoch Schonlein purpura
- Behcet's disease

Some cases of epididymitis are idiopathic.

Clinical features

Sexual history is extremely important. Symptoms are variable. Pain and swelling usually begin in the tail (lowermost part) of the epididymis. Other features are scrotal erythema, fever and chills with or without dysuria. There may be associated orchitis. Inflammatory markers are elevated, and if untreated, epididymitis can lead to abscess formation and rarely to septicaemia, especially in the immunocompromised patients.

Differential diagnosis

- testicular torsion
- torsion of hydatid of Morgagni
- testicular tumours

Investigations

Urethral swabs for Chlamydia and *N. gonorrhoeae* should be obtained as well as urine culture and sensitivity, urethral smear for Grams stain, and midstream urine for immunofluorescence. Molecular methods using ligase chain reaction or polymerase chain reaction have high sensitivity for Chlamydia. Colour Doppler imaging may be useful, especially to distinguish between acute epididymitis and testicular torsion.

Management

- bed rest
- scrotal support
- analgesia
- non-steroidal anti-inflammatory drugs (NSAIDs).
- antibiotics

For sexually acquired infections, doxycycline 100 mg b.d. × 14 days or equivalent should be given.

For non-sexually acquired infections, ciprofloxacin 500 mg b.d. × 14 days may be prescribed. Where there is potential overlap with chlamydial and bacterial agents, levofloxacin 500 mg o.d. × 14 days or ofloxacin 200 mg o.d. × 14 days may be given.

If culture results indicate gonococcal infection, ceftriaxone should be added. In sexually acquired cases, once confirmed, it is important to treat the partners and contacts as well.

If urinary tract tuberculosis (TB) is identified, a full course of anti-tuberculous treatment is indicated with appropriate screening of contacts as well as investigation of the patient's respiratory tract.

Complications

- residual pain and discomfort
- abscess formation
- testicular ischaemia and infarction
- chronic epididymitis and pain
- infertility.

Further reading

Cole FL, Vogler R. The acute, non-traumatic scrotum: assessment, diagnosis and management. J Am Acad Nurse Pract 2004;16(2):50–6.

Kodner C. Sexually transmitted infections in men. Prim Care 2003;30(1):173–91.

Hagley M. Epididymo-orchitis and epididymitis: review of causes and management of unusual forms. Int J STD AIDS 2003;14(6):373–7.

Erectile dysfunction

Richard Pearcy

The inability to maintain an erection sufficient for intercourse is a common problem. As many as 30–40% of the British male population may suffer from it. Both the incidence and prevalence increase with age. Traditionally, erectile dysfunction (ED) has been subdivided into psychogenic or organic (neurological, hormonal and vascular). However, the majority of patients probably have a combination of both and with modern treatment the distinction is not required. Risk factors include diabetes mellitus (and how well it is controlled), hypertension, heart disease, hypercholesterolaemia, smoking, major pelvic surgery and some drugs (e.g. β-blockers).

Investigations

These may include testosterone, follicle stimulating hormone (FSH), luteinizing hormone (LH), prolactin, fasting lipid profile and glucose, prostate specific antigen (PSA) and blood pressure measurement. Testosterone, FSH and LH are included to look for testicular failure and prolactin to detect a pituitary adenoma. ED has been shown to be closely related to vascular disease, so it seems sensible to assess the patient's lipid profile, glucose level and blood pressure.

Treatments

Phosphodiesterase inhibitors

Phosphodiesterase (PDE-5) inhibitors include tadalafil, vardenafil and sildenafil. All these drugs inhibit PDE-5 (the enzyme responsible for cGMP breakdown), thereby potentiating the effect of the natural vasodilator nitric oxide in the penile vasculature. All the available drugs are similar; however, some differences exist. Tadalafil has a long half-life (17 hours), allowing administration long before the required intercourse, and has the possibility of enabling frequent acts during the time that the therapeutic level is achieved. Tadalafil, and to a lesser extent vardenafil, do not have to be taken on an empty stomach. However, all members of this group of drugs has a significant interaction with nitrates. The concomitant administration may lead to a substantial fall in blood pressure.

Centrally acting drugs

Apomorphine acts on the paraventricular nucleus of the hypothalamus, potentiating parasympathetic outflow to the spinal cord. This drug, although less effective than PDE-5 inhibitors, has the advantage of not interacting with nitrates. Apomorphine has been used as an emetic, but at the dose used for ED, nausea does not seem to be a large problem. The commonest side effect reported was yawning.

Intra-urethral medicated urethral system for erections (MUSE)

This system delivers, via a specially designed applicator, a pellet containing prostaglandin E1 (PGE1) to the urethra. The arrangement of the penile vasculature is such that enough of the active drug enters the corpus cavernosum so that vasodilatation (via cAMP) takes place. Some patients receive benefit from this system.

Hormone therapy

If the level of testosterone has been shown to be low, a therapeutic trial of testosterone administration may be worthwhile. However, the relationship between erections and testosterone is not clearly defined, and testosterone delivery can be difficult (intra-muscular injections, patches or implants). Before embarking on testosterone administration, a rectal examination and PSA level test are recommended as testosterone may make an undiagnosed prostate cancer grow rapidly. There is no good evidence that boosting normal hormone levels will improve erections.

Intracavernosal injections

Intracavernosal injection is the most effective ED treatment. The delivery system (a variety are marketed) using a fine-bore needle delivers PGE1 directly to the corpus cavernosum. Disadvantages to this treatment are that it is invasive and requires skilled training and commitment by the patient. If this treatment fails to achieve an erection at maximum dose, a surgical implant is likely to be the next option.

Vacuum devices

Vacuum devices act by drawing blood into the penis and a constriction band is applied to the base to stop venous outflow. Disadvantages are that it leads to a cold 'unrealistic' penis, but for those patients who like this therapy it has the advantage of being cheap after the initial outlay.

Surgical options

Penile implants are available in two types, malleable and inflatable. Only malleable prostheses are generally available on the NHS, but they are semi-rigid and do not mimic the natural situation. Inflatable prostheses have a high degree of patient and partner satisfaction, provide a 'normal' feeling penis, are easy to use, but they can fail, are more expensive and carry a significant infective incidence.

Further reading

Melman A, Gingell JC. The epidemiology and pathophysiology of erectile dysfunction (review). J Urol 1999;161(1):5–11.

Genital dermatoses

Venkat Gudi

Lichen simplex

Introduction

Persistent itching and scratching can result in thickening of genital skin with accentuation of skin markings. This is called lichen simplex chronicus. Its aetiology is unknown, although in many patients a personal or family history of atopy can be elicited. Use of local irritants, contact allergy and psychological factors may all play a role in a self-perpetuating itch–scratch cycle. It generally occurs on accessible areas of genital skin, especially the labia majora in women and the scrotum in men. The perianal region is another commonly affected site.

Presentation

People give a history of itch. On examination, one can see localized areas of thickened skin with prominent natural skin creases, hyperpigmentation and excoriation.

Diagnosis

A clinical diagnoisis is usually sufficient and a skin biopsy can be limited to those patients in whom the diagnosis is in doubt.

Treatment

This is a good point to mention the risk of atrophy and striae formation when using potent topical steroids on genital skin. Topical steroids increase in potency if applied under occlusion and with increase of local body temperature. This is especially true in the genital region where body folds and clothes provide a strong occlusive effect. Maintenance treatment of any inflammatory dermatosis in the genital region should be limited to mild and moderate strength topical steroids (e.g. 1% hydrocortisone ointment and clobetasone butyrate 0.05% or Eumovate ointment) and patients should be advised to use the minimum amount necessary for relief of symptoms. The risk of cutaneous side effects with topical steroids is greatest with very strong topical steroids, e.g. clobetasol propionate 0.05% (Dermovate), and so its use should be under specialist supervision only. Potent topical steroids e.g. betamethasone valerate 0.1% (Betnovate) can be used in acute inflammatory disease, but should be limited to 2 weeks at a time. It must be explained to patients that they can step down on the strength of topical steroid once symptoms improve.

Emollients are also a useful adjunct to the treatment of lichen simplex. Both ointment-based (Epaderm, 50:50 white soft paraffin in liquid paraffin) and cream-based (Diprobase, aqueous cream) formulations are available. The choice of emollient depends on the dryness of the skin and patient preference. Ointments are more effective but are cumbersome to use.

The inflammation of lichen simplex can be countered by use of potent topical steroids of moderate strength, e.g. Betnovate daily for 2 weeks. An ointment-based emollient should also be used such as Epaderm. Sedative antihistamines, e.g hydroxyzine and chlorpheniramine are beneficial since the itch is often worse at night. Doxepin, a tricyclic antidepressant, is another useful drug to help itch at a dose of 25–100 mg at night. All usual precautions concerning use of antihistamines and tricyclic antidepressants should be observed.

Patients who do not respond to the above treatment should be referred to a dermatologist or GUM physician, where more potent topical steroids, intralesional steroids or surgery can be considered. Some areas have special clinics for people with vulval or penile dermatoses.

Other management
General measures for pruritus of any cause should be followed (see page 33, Genital itch). Many patients with lichen simplex may have used a variety of topical agents in an attempt to get relief of itch. If this is the case, contact allergy might be contributing to the symptoms and hence detailed patch testing is advisable. Avoidance of proven sensitisers may help to ameliorate symptoms.

Further reading
Lynch PJ. Lichen simplex chronicus (atopic/neurodermatitis) of the anogenital region. Dermatol Ther 2004;17(1):8–19.

Intertrigo

Introduction
Intertrigo is inflammation of the folds of the skin. This is usually due to chafing or infection associated with occlusion and moisture, especially in obese patients. It can also be due to primary skin diseases such as psoriasis or seborrheic dermatitis. Autoimmune or inherited blistering diseases such as pemphigus vulgaris or Hailey–Hailey disease, respectively, can also manifest in this region.

Presentation
The patient complains of itch. In mild cases the skin creases are merely red but in severe cases pain, ulceration and discharge can occur.

Complications
The lesions can get secondarily infected, with resultant change in morphology.

Diagnosis
Management of severe intertrigo will need an accurate diagnosis, which in some patients means a biopsy. If there is copious discharge, a swab should be taken for bacteriology and virology.

Treatment

If there is a lot of discharge, potassium permanganate soaks should be applied. This solution can be made up at a strength of 0.01% from dissolving one tablet of Permitabs in 4 litres of lukewarm water. An application for 15–20 minutes twice daily helps reduce discharge.

If superinfection is suspected, a broad-spectrum antibiotic covering both Gram-positive and Gram-negative organisms is necessary, e.g. co-amoxiclav. If herpes is suspected, aciclovir can be started in appropriate doses. If it is thought to be due to dermatitis, topical steroids are helpful.

It is important to use the appropriate strength of topical steroids in anogenital inflammatory disease. For short-term use (less than 2 weeks) a potent topical steroid can be used if disease is severe, e.g. Betnovate®. It is advisable to change to a weaker steroid, e.g. Eumovate® or hydrocortisone after this period; longer use of potent topical steroids is associated with marked skin thinning and striae. If fungal infection is suspected, it is important to avoid topical steroids as rapid spread of rash can occur.

Tinea cruris

Introduction

Tinea cruris is a commonly occurring dermatophyte infection of skin in the inguinal and anogenital region. It occurs almost exclusively in males, is associated commonly with fungal infection in toe- or fingernails, and spreads gradually, especially if topical steroids are applied.

Presentation

Symptoms are characterized by severe itch and a spreading rash. The typical rash of tinea is annular with a scaly border and central clearing. Topical steroid application will rapidly change this morphology and the rash may look very atypical.

Complications

Topical steroids can make the infection go deeper in the skin, resulting in folliculitis.

Diagnosis

It is useful to confirm the diagnosis of tinea first before starting specific treatment.

A diagnosis is easily made by sending skin scrapings from the edge of the lesion for microscopy using potassium hydroxide, and fungal culture.

Treatment

Treatment with topical antifungals like miconazole and terbinafine are curative for tinea cruris. A 4–6 week course of twice daily application of antifungal cream is the usual regimen.

Other management

Tinea can recur and this should be explained to patients. It is important to deal with reservoir sites such as the nails with oral antifungal medication (terbinafine or itraconazole) to reduce the chances of recurrence. Keeping the groin dry is also a useful measure in prevention.

Sexual contacts
Tinea cruris is not sexually transmitted.

Psoriasis

Introduction
Psoriasis can occur anywhere in the anogenital region, but commonly affects the intertriginous regions, i.e. groin folds and intergluteal folds.

Presentation
Genital psoriasis is characterized by erythematous rash with a clear border, associated with maceration and erosion of tissues. Scaling, a classic feature of psoriasis elsewhere, is usually absent.

Complications
None if it remains localized to genital skin.

Diagnosis
Diagnosis is usually based on clinical features. Biopsy is not always helpful as typical histological features of psoriasis are absent in intertriginous areas.

Treatments
Many of the treatments used for psoriasis elsewhere on the body such as coal tar, dithranol and calcipotriol are too irritant for use in intertriginous areas. Topical steroids are usually the only agents helpful in this situation. Use of a medium- to low-potency topical steroid is advisable (e.g. Eumovate) to reduce the risk of steroid side effects.

Contact dermatitis

Introduction
Allergic or irritant contact dermatitis of the anogenital region is usually acute, but chronic contact dermatitis can occur.

In men, common allergens include rubber antioxidants or accelerators in condoms, lanolin in creams, topical anaesthetic agents, male and female contraceptives, and feminine hygiene products (with which the patient may have come in contact during sexual intercourse). Natural latex protein is the allergen in latex sensitivity, which causes a type I reaction with urticaria and angioedema.

In women, vulvar dermatitis or pruritus is often (in more than 50% of patients) associated with contact allergy, usually to medications or vehicles used in their preparation: lanolin in creams, propylene glycol in KY jelly and topical anaesthetic agents in some preparations promoted for relief of anogenital pruritus. Other common allergens include fragrances and nickel.

In both sexes, irritant contact dermatitis can result from overzealous 'cleaning' using powerful detergents or by application of a variety of toxic substances in high concentration to skin.

Presentation
Erythema, itch and blistering are the usual symptoms. In men, the foreskin can become oedematous. Distribution of the rash depends on its aetiology; it can spread easily to involve the shaft of the penis, scrotal skin and the inner thighs.

Latex allergy to rubber condoms usually manifests acutely with massive foreskin swelling within minutes of contact. The patient may give a prior history of urticarial reaction to rubber products such as balloons and gloves.

Chronic allergic contact dermatitis is usually suggested by a history of burning, stinging or aggravation of pre-existing rash after applying the offending allergen. However, in many patients, no such history is available.

Diagnosis
Diagnosis is suggested by the above clinical features, but clarification needs detailed patch testing with a large number of standard and accessory allergens and should include testing for allergy to the alleged products 'as is'. This is generally performed in an outpatient clinic setting in dermatology.

Treatment
Contact allergy to rubber may be severe in some patients, so much so that they will have to use condoms made of other materials like polyurethane (Avanti®) or lamb caecum. The diagnosis of latex allergy needs confirmation by appropriate skin prick testing, as this has implications for the patients' occupation and clinical care. Careful avoidance of allergens along with prudent use of moderately potent topical steroids will result in improvement in symptoms in the majority of patients.

Anogenital lichen sclerosus

Introduction
Lichen sclerosus (LS) is a common, chronic inflammatory condition usually seen in the anogenital region. Women are affected six times more commonly than men, usually between the ages of 50 and 59. It can affect other areas of skin in about 10% of patients with anogenital LS. Its precise aetiology is unclear, but LS can be associated with a variety of autoimmune diseases.

LS of the glans penis was formerly known as balanitis xerotica obliterans.

Presentation
In women, symptoms include severe itch and soreness of the vulval and perianal region. They may also complain of dysuria, dyspareunia and pain on defecation. Painful fissures and tears may occur with sexual intercourse and following defecation. In many patients, the condition may remain essentially asymptomatic and signs may be noted on routine examination. In women, LS can affect the perineum, labia majora, fourchette and clitoris leading to a figure-of-eight shape on examination.

Skin and/or mucosa becomes pale and shiny. Haemorrhage under the skin or mucosa is a striking feature of LS. Advanced, untreated LS can present with severe scarring with narrowing of the introitus and resorption of the labia minora as well as the clitoris.

Men share many symptoms such as itch and soreness of penile mucosa and skin as well as traumatic fissures, especially after sexual intercourse.

LS can occur in prepubertal children and signs may be confused with sexual abuse. Careful history and examination will usually lead to the correct diagnosis.

Complications

LS is a scarring process and in women it may result in progressive narrowing of the vaginal introitus with consequent sexual problems. In men, it can tighten the foreskin leading to phimosis and can narrow the urethral meatus causing poor flow and back-pressure, potentially resulting in renal failure.

> About 5% of women with LS may develop a **squamous cell carcinoma** in the affected area. It is important that patients are aware of this risk and that non-healing areas are biopsied to exclude malignancy. It is not known whether treated LS poses the same risk as untreated LS.

Diagnosis

Confirmatory skin or mucosal biopsy is necessary in most patients because other conditions such as lichen planus and mucosal pemphigoid can mimic LS.

Treatment

Management of LS is aimed at improvement of symptoms, detection and management of complications, and monitoring for occurrence of malignancy. As yet, there is no cure for LS and treatment is generally of long duration; this fact should be explained to patients.

Potent topical steroids have been shown to be very effective in relieving symptoms of LS. Clobetasol propionate 0.05% (Dermovate®) ointment once daily for 3 months, then gradually reduced to once a week, is a suitable regimen to achieve control of LS. A 30-g tube of Dermovate® should last about 6 months, achieving adequate control of LS. With treatment, the pallor of anogenital skin and symptoms should improve significantly; severe scarring is unlikely to resolve.

A few patients may not respond to topical steroids. Treatment is difficult in this group; there are recent reports of the efficacy of topical tacrolimus 0.1% ointment in such cases, but this treatment is best undertaken under specialist supervision.

Circumcision will be needed in complicated LS with severe irreversible phimosis. Meatotomy is also sometimes needed if the external urethral meatus is narrowed as a result of scarring. Surgical management in women should be limited to correction of a very narrow introitus leading to difficulties with micturition or sexual intercourse. LS tends to spread to areas of trauma and so it is important to control the condition medically, before proceeding to surgery.

Lichen planus

Lichen planus (LP) is an inflammatory disorder of skin and mucous membranes with characteristic clinical and histological features. It can affect genital mucosa or skin either as part of generalized lichen planus or more uncommonly, this region can be the only location affected. Rarely, an LP-like rash can be seen as a result of allergy to drugs.

Presentation

LP can present in two ways on genital mucosa: as an asymptomatic reticulate (net-like) violaceous rash or more rarely as an eroded area. The latter is extremely painful.

Diagnosis

LP can usually be diagnosed on clinical grounds, but erosive LP often needs histo-logical confirmation because other blistering diseases such as pemphigus or erythema multiforme can present in a similar fashion.

Treatment

If the patient is asymptomatic, no active treatment is necessary except to reassure the patient. The course of the disease generally lasts about 2–3 years before it sponta-neously clears. If painful erosions are a feature, it is important to examine other mucosal surfaces to classify the disease. Often, superpotent topical steroids like Dermovate ointment are used; many patients with erosive LP often need a course of oral prednisolone to achieve healing. It is important to consider drugs as a possible contributor to the rash; close correlation of drug history and onset of rash should make it easy to identify the culprit drug.

Genital tract pre-malignancy (genital intra-epithelial neoplasia)

Sarah Wallage

Genital squamous cell cancers have a pre-invasive stage of intra-epithelial neoplasia. The likelihood and timescale of progression is better understood for cervical disease than for vulval, vaginal, penile and anal intra-epithelial neoplasia. Pre-invasive lesions are often asymptomatic and even symptomatic external disease may have a non-specific appearance causing delayed diagnosis. Screening and treatment of pre-invasive lesions may prevent progression to malignancy but do have associated physical and psychological morbidity and economic costs.

Intra-epithelial neoplasia is more frequent and progression to invasive disease accelerated among people who are immune suppressed. Immune suppression may be associated with HIV infection or prescribed drugs such as azathioprine or cyclosporin following an organ transplant or for autoimmune disease. Squamous cell cervical carcinoma is an AIDS-defining disease. Cigarette smoking damages the local mucosal immune response by affecting Langerhans cell function. Giving up smoking may encourage regression of low-grade intra-epithelial neoplasia. Highly active antiretroviral therapy (HAART) may be expected to reduce the prevalence of intra-epithelial neoplasia in people with HIV. This has not been confirmed, although there is a suggestion that cervical intra-epithelial neoplasia (CIN) is more likely to regress with successful HAART than is anal intra-epithelial neoplasia (AIN).

Human papilloma virus (HPV) infection is associated with all types of genital intra-epithelial neoplasia. Genital HPV infection is very common; it is estimated that 80% of the sexually active population will be infected at some time in their life, but infection is usually transient and subclinical. More than 130 HPV types have been described so far. Genital warts are usually caused by HPV 6 and 11 (see page 187). Persistence of certain HPV types, particularly types 16, 18, 31, 33 and 35, is associated with malignant disease.

HPV vaccines are at an advanced stage of development and have potential for both prevention and treatment of malignant disease.

Genital warts often respond well to the topical immunity-enhancing drug imiquimod (Aldara^R). Results for imiquimod treatment of intra-epithelial neoplasia have been mixed and disappointing with high rates of recurrence and drop out due to discomfort.

Trials of topical 5-fluorouracil, an antimetabolite, have had similar findings with treatment often limited by side effects. Topical cidofovir, an antiviral drug, is undergoing trials.

Intra-epithelial neoplasia can be multifocal, e.g. women with vulval intra-epithelial neoplasia have an increased risk of cervical disease. Discovery of disease in one site should lead to examination of the whole lower genital tract.

Histologically, intra-epithelial neoplasia can be divided into low grade/stage I and high grade/stage II to III lesions. In low-grade disease, dysplasia is seen only in the lower third of the epithelium nearest the basement membrane. In high-grade disease, dysplasia extends to the middle or upper third. Dysplastic changes include epithelial proliferation, loss of architecture and atypical squamous cells with increased nuclear:cytoplasmic ratio and mitotic figures.

Cervical intra-epithelial neoplasia

CIN arises at the squamocolumnar junction and is asymptomatic. The position of the squamocolumnar junction alters during puberty, pregnancy and at the menopause. Squamous metaplasia is the term to describe changes in which columnar epithelium reverts to squamous type. This 'tidal area' is called the transformation zone.

> There is clear evidence that squamous cell cervical carcinoma is preceded by CIN, and the national cervical cytology screening programme has developed to detect high-grade CIN and to allow treatment before malignant change occurs. It is estimated that 40% of women with high-grade CIN would develop carcinoma over 10 years if untreated. Low-grade disease, however, has a 50% chance of spontaneous regression. Cervical adenocarcinoma may be detected incidentally, but the screening programme is not designed for this.

In the UK, women are offered cervical cytology tests, or 'smears', every 3 years from age 25–49 and every 5 years from age 50–64. The recommended frequency and age limits changed in 2004 and differ in Scotland. There is a national screening service involving primary and secondary care and auditing practice and outcomes. Liquid-based cytology techniques have a lower rate of inadequate tests and fewer screener errors than previous spatula and slide methods.

Cervical smears sample the transformation zone and aim to detect cytological dyskaryosis as a marker for CIN. Approximately 8% of all smears will show dyskaryosis. The chance of high-grade CIN increases from 40% in women with a mildly dyskaryotic smear to 90% with severe dyskaryosis. Cervical cytology is not 100% sensitive and may be reported as normal in the presence of CIN or carcinoma.

Cervical carcinoma is extremely rare in women under 25, whereas transient CIN is common. This is likely to be related to a newly sexually acquired HPV infection. Delaying onset of cytological screening until age 20–25 aims to avoid unnecessary overtreatment. New CIN in women over 50 with a full negative screening history is rare, so screening frequency can be reduced. In the future, testing for high-risk HPV types may help rationalize management of women with abnormal cytology. For example, women with negative smears until age 50 who are also negative for HPV 16 and 18 may be discharged from cytology recall, or women with low-grade CIN and negative HPV testing may be able to avoid immediate colposcopy.

Colposcopy is indicated if the cervix looks suspicious, if cytology has shown dyskaryosis or if three smears have been inadequate for diagnosis or have shown borderline abnormality. Colposcopy involves examination of the cervix with a ×20 power microscope. Application of 3% acetic acid and Lugol's iodine can highlight areas of dysplasia. The whole transformation zone must be seen for colposcopy to be adequate. This may be impossible after treatment or in post-menopausal women. Colposcopy is not 100% sensitive or specific. Directed biopsy can be taken for histological examination if the degree of dysplasia is unclear, or excision biopsy can be performed when cytology, colposcopy or biopsy suggest high-grade squamous lesions.

Excision biopsy or large loop excision of the transformation zone (LLETZ) is usually performed under local anaesthetic using diathermy. Lasers have been used but require special equipment and have no clear treatment advantage. LLETZ removes the transformation zone to a depth of 7 mm and aims to completely excise the lesion as well as providing a specimen for histological assessment. A standard LLETZ procedure does not affect subsequent pregnancy or delivery.

Cervical cytology follow-up is needed after treatment for CIN as disease may not have been completely excised, and treated women still have a higher risk of recurrent CIN or carcinoma than other women. Persistent abnormal cytology with inadequate colposcopy after LLETZ is an indication for a deeper excision cone biopsy or hysterectomy. Glandular abnormalities detected by cytology need different management approaches, including deep, extended LLETZ or knife cone and endometrial assessment.

Vulval intra-epithelial neoplasia

Vulval intra-epithelial neoplasia (VIN) may present in any age group and has a wide clinical spectrum. Women may complain of itching or soreness or be asymptomatic. Raised nodules, velvety plaques, erythema or hyperpigmentation may be seen on examination. Lesions may be multifocal or unifocal. Some women present after unsuccessful treatment of 'warts' or 'thrush' or with 'healing problems' at an old episiotomy scar. Women with lichen sclerosus et atrophicus are at increased risk of vulval carcinoma and any persistent fissure, ulcer or plaque must be biopsied to exclude new VIN or frank neoplastic change.

Clinical diagnosis is not exact and even high-grade VIN may cause few symptoms.

Any vulval lesion, whether symptomatic or just noticed on examination should be biopsied and sent for histological assessment. This can be performed simply in clinic with local anaesthetic injection and a 3- to 4-mm punch biopsy. Haemostasis is readily achieved with silver nitrate or an absorbable suture.

Low-grade lesions may be managed conservatively by 6 monthly review, but high-grade lesions are now thought to have a 10–20% risk of malignant progression and should be excised. Input from plastic surgeons may be needed to optimize cosmetic and functional results.

Laser vaporization has been used to treat large areas of VIN by ablation to 1 mm depth in non-hairy areas and to 2.5 mm in hairy areas. Multiple biopsies are essential to exclude malignancy before ablation.

Paget's disease is a form of intra-epithelial neoplasia arising from apocrine glands, which may be detected on vulval biopsy. It has malignant potential, is often multi-focal and frequently recurs despite wide, full-thickness local excision.

Vaginal intra-epithelial neoplasia

Vaginal intra-epithelial neoplasia (VaIN) is a rare condition usually found in the upper vagina at colposcopy for women who are known to have CIN or VIN. Incidence is increased after pelvic radiotherapy.

VaIN may develop after hysterectomy for squamous cell cervical carcinoma and can occur in the vault suture line making detection difficult. Colposcopic assessment of the vagina as well as of the cervix is needed before hysterectomy for CIN/squamous carcinoma to guide excision of any coexisting VaIN.

Low-grade VaIN may regress, but high-grade VaIN is thought to have a 10–15% risk of progression to carcinoma and is generally treated by excision. Laser vaporization may be used for widespread or multifocal lesions once malignancy has been excluded by multiple biopsies. Plastic surgery techniques and reconstructive procedures may be needed depending on the site and extent of disease.

Clear cell vaginal adenocarcinoma is a separate rare condition with increased incidence in daughters of women who took diethylstilboestrol (DES) during pregnancy. These women may have cervical and uterine anatomical abnormalities. DES treatment to prevent miscarriage was stopped in the early 1970s, and affected daughters usually present in their 20s, so new cases are becoming rarer.

Penile intra-epithelial neoplasia

Penile intra-epithelial neoplasia (PIN) is probably underdiagnosed and plaque-type lesions may be inadvertently treated as genital warts. Studies have found PIN more frequently in partners of women with CIN. The average age of men with stage III PIN is 7 years older than men with stage I PIN, suggesting some progression over time. However, penile cancer remains a rare condition (1.4 per 100 000 men), so some regression is also likely. Treatment of high-grade disease is by excision. Surgery and laser treatment have been used.

Erythroplasia of Queyrat and Bowen's disease can present as scarlet plaques and have a risk of malignant change. As with vulval disease, persistent skin changes on the penis must be biopsied under local anaesthetic to establish a diagnosis (plain lidocaine without adrenaline).

Anal intra-epithelial neoplasia

Anal carcinoma is a rare condition but with a much higher incidence in the immuno-suppressed, particularly men who have sex with men (80 per 100 000 in HIV-positive gay men compared with 1 per 100 000 in the whole population).

High-grade anal intra-epithelial neoplasia (AIN) has been found in 10% of HIV-positive gay men who have CD4 counts of less than 200 with an estimated 1 in 200 risk of progression to anal squamous cell carcinoma per annum in this group. Risk of progression for other patient groups is less clear.

Some patients with AIN may have pruritus, soreness or visible changes. Changes develop at the squamocolumnar junction, so proctoscopy is necessary for examination up to the white line of Hilton. A ×20 microscope and application of 3% acetic acid and Lugol's iodine have been found to identify lesions, as for colposcopy. Exfoliative anal cytology using a cotton bud can show dyskaryosis in a similar way to cervical cytology. The sensitivity and specificity of the test are still being established. Anal cytology may be useful to screen high-risk groups but is not widely used.

High-grade or symptomatic disease is treated by excision, with care to avoid sphincter damage.

Gonorrhoea

Steve Baguley

Introduction

Gonorrhoea is caused by the Gram-negative diplococcus *Neisseria gonorrhoeae*. In the UK, the various conditions caused by the bacterium declined in incidence throughout the 1980s and into the early 1990s, but since 1994 it has become more common. In 2002 there were about 26 000 cases diagnosed at Genitourinary Medicine clinics in the UK. An unknown number of people were diagnosed in other settings. The increase in cases is thought to be due to increased sexual activity, in particular, more people having concurrent sexual partners.

The disease is most common in large cities and in areas of relative deprivation. Condoms are effective in preventing transmission of gonorrhoea, but they need to be used for fellatio as well as vaginal and anal sex since pharyngeal infection is not uncommon and is usually asymptomatic.

The bacteria can infect any mucosal surface, including the conjunctiva, cervix, urethra, pharynx and rectum.

The pathophysiology of *N. gonorrhoeae* and the relative virulence of different subtypes depend on the antigenic characteristics of their respective surface proteins. Certain subtypes are able to evade serum immune responses and are more likely to lead to disseminated infection. Plasmid and non-plasmid genes are transmitted between different subtypes. It is the exchange of surface protein genes that results in high host susceptibility to reinfection.

Presentation

The etymology of gonorrhoea is from the Greek *gonos:* semen and *rhoia:* flow. Anyone who has seen a man with the typical heavy urethral discharge of gonorrhoea will know how it got its name. But urethral discharge is not universal – 10% of men with urethral infection are asymptomatic at that site, although they may have signs of infection when examined.

Since *N. gonorrhoeae* can infect so many sites, people with the condition can present to a variety of healthcare providers. Table 1 shows the possible modes of (symptomatic) presentation, with the more common presentations listed first.

Table 1 Symptoms of gonorrhoea

Sex	Site	Possible symptoms	Comment
Men	Urethral infection	White/yellow/green often heavy urethral discharge Dysuria	90% of cases
	Scrotal contents	Unilateral scrotal pain and swelling	If epididymo-orchitis. Do not confuse with testicular torsion!
Women (asymptomatic in 50% of cases)	Genital	Abnormal vaginal discharge	Commonest single symptom
		Dysuria	Unusual, as is symptomatic urethral discharge
		Intermenstrual bleeding/ post-coital bleeding	Less common a symptom than in Chlamydia
	Abdomen	Pelvic pain	If pelvic inflammatory disease (PID) or if chorioamnionitis
		Right upper quadrant pain	If perihepatitis, aka Fitz–Hugh–Curtis syndrome
Both sexes	Pharynx	Sore throat, dysphagia	Almost always asymptomatic
	Anus/rectum	Anorectal pain, rectal discharge	Usually asymptomatic. In women, rectal infection can occur by spread from the vagina as well as by anal sex
	Eyes	Purulent eye in neonate or adult	Conjunctivitis is usually bilateral in neonates but unilateral in adults. Can lead to blindness if left untreated
	Musculoskeletal	Single large joint arthritis (usually a knee) with severe pain, oedema, erythema and decreased range of movement	A common cause of septic arthritis in young people
		Migratory polyarthralgia and polyarthritis with pain, tenderness, decreased range of motion, and erythema	Rare. A feature of disseminated gonococcal infection (DGI)
		Tenosynovitis usually of the hands	Rare. A feature of DGI
		Muscle abscess presenting as localized tenderness, oedema and pain	Rare. A feature of DGI
	Central nervous system	Meningism/meningitis	Rare. A feature of DGI. Progresses less rapidly than meningococcal meningitis
	Cardiovascular system	Murmur, tachycardia and other symptoms/signs of endocarditis	Rare. A feature of DGI
	Systemic	Fever usually $<39°C$	Rare. A feature of DGI and severe PID
	Skin	Maculopapular, vesico-pustular or necrotic rash. Usually occurring on the torso, limbs, palms and soles.	Rare. Seen in DGI. Usually spares the head. Lesions are usually at different stages of development at presentation

Complications

Women

As with chlamydia, serious complications are more common in women than in men. Infection can ascend from the cervix leading to pelvic inflammatory disease (PID). This can cause pelvic pain and in severe cases, peritonitis. Late complications include chronic abdominal pain, ectopic pregnancy and infertility (see PID, page 152). Chorioamnionitis can lead to miscarriage and pre-term labour.

Men

Spread from the urethra can cause epididymo-orchitis (see epididymo-orchitis, page 99) and occasionally prostatitis (see prostatitis, page 159). Urethral strictures can occur following inflammation and scarring of the periurethral glands. This can occasionally lead to urethral obstruction and infertility. The mythical 'cocktail umbrella' device feared by many first-time male GU clinic attendees probably has its origin in the devices used to treat urethral strictures.

Both sexes

In about 1% of cases, infection can spread haematogenously to distant sites leading to disseminated gonococcal infection (DGI). This has numerous manifestations (see Table 1), although the most common symptom is joint or tendon pain. Later complications include permanent neurologic sequelae from meningitis and destruction of heart valves by endocarditis.

DGI is more common in women and appears to be facilitated by menstruation. Untreated conjunctivitis can lead to corneal scarring, globe perforation and blindness. Gonococcal septic arthritis can cause joint destruction, although this is less common than in septic arthritis of other causes, e.g. staphylococcal.

Gonorrhoea increases the chance of acquiring or transmitting HIV from an episode of unprotected sex.

Fetus and neonate

Infections in pregnant women can lead to miscarriage and prematurity. Neonatal infection can cause symptoms at any site but most commonly conjunctivitis. Rarely generalized sepsis or DGI can occur.

Diagnosis

- Specimens should be collected from all sites where the infection is suspected. In men, this usually means the urethra unless they have had sex with men, in which case it is customary to take rectal and pharyngeal specimens too, depending on the sexual history.
- In women, the main site to sample is the cervix, although the pharynx and rectum should be sampled if there are symptoms at those sites or as indicated by the sexual history. A urethral swab is useful if the woman is a contact of gonorrhoea or if you are working somewhere where gonorrhoea is relatively common.

- Which diagnostic method(s) you use will depend on where you are working.
- The mainstay of diagnosis remains culture, which has a sensitivity of around 95%. Swabs are plated onto selective, enriched media (e.g. chocolate agar) and growth of oxidase-positive, Gram-negative diplococci confirms the diagnosis. *N. gonorrhoeae* requires a CO_2-enriched atmosphere.
- In most GUM clinics, swabs are plated in the consultation room, but sending a swab to the lab in transport medium gives acceptable results. If the interval between specimen collection and plating is greater than 12 hours, the sensitivity starts to fall.
- Gram-stained microscopy can speed diagnosis and this is a sensitive and specific test in male urethral specimens. In female urethral specimens and samples from other sites, it is much less useful because of the presence of other bacteria with similar morphology.
- If you suspect gonorrhoea, smear some of the specimen onto a slide, air dry it and send to the lab. If the organism fails to grow, the diagnosis might then be made from microscopy.
- Nucleic acid amplification tests (which can use urine as a specimen) are available but are not widely used in the UK. In low-prevalence populations they generate a lot of false positives. Culture is still necessary in positive cases to confirm the diagnosis and determine antibiotic sensitivity.
- In the absence of laboratory tests, a clinical diagnosis can usually be made in men with classic symptoms and signs, but this should always be confirmed if at all possible.
- If DGI is suspected, blood and joint effusions should be sent for Gram stain and culture, although negative stain results and sterile cultures do not rule out the condition.
- Cerebrospinal fluid should be stained and cultured if there are signs or symptoms of meningitis.
- Gram stains and cultures of genital, rectal, conjunctival and pharyngeal secretions also should be obtained when DGI is suspected, even if the patient has no localized symptoms at any of those sites.

Treatment

Treatment is complicated by the high proportion of isolates that are resistant to antibiotics. Well-characterized plasmids commonly carry antibiotic-resistance genes, most notably penicillinase. The exchange of antibiotic resistance genes has led to extremely high levels of resistance to beta-lactam antibiotics over the last two decades. More recently, fluoroquinolone resistance also has been documented on multiple continents.

In the UK, ciprofloxacin and penicillin are now inappropriate for blind treatment of gonorrhoea due to high levels of resistance. Of course, if sensitivity results are available you can choose any agent on the list the microbiology lab give you.

- blind treatment of suspected/confirmed uncomplicated anogenital gonorrhoea:
  - cefixime 400 mg p.o. once (first choice), or
  - ceftriaxone 250 mg i.m. once, or

- cefotaxime 500 mg i.m. once.
- if sensitivities known:
  - ciprofloxacin 500 mg p.o. once (not if pregnant, breast feeding or under 5), or
  - ofloxacin 400 mg p.o. once (not if pregnant, breast feeding or under 5), or
  - amoxicillin 3 g p.o. once plus probenecid 1 g p.o. once.
- spectinomycin 2 g i.m. once is useful for treating quinolone- and penicillin-resistant cases in people who are allergic to cephalosporins. Unfortunately it can be hard to obtain
- amoxicillin and spectinomycin are less effective at eradicating pharyngeal infection than other agents
- treatment of gonococcal pelvic inflammatory disease – see page 155
- treatment of gonococcal epididymo-orchitis – see page 100
- treatment of DGI – admit to hospital and exclude endocarditis and meningitis
- dermatitis/arthritis:
  - ceftriaxone 1 g i.v. o.d., or
  - cefotaxime 1 g i.v. t.d.s. until symptoms improve for 24 hours, then
  - cefixime 400 mg p.o. o.d. (or other agent if sensitivities known) to extend treatment to a total of 7 days
  - plus repeated joint aspiration if large joint septic arthritis.
- endocarditis – ceftriaxone 2 g i.v. b.d. for 4 weeks
- meningitis – ceftriaxone 2 g i.v. b.d. for 4 weeks
- conjunctivitis (adult)
  - ceftriaxone 1 g i.m. or i.v. once (and lavage with saline)
  - if deep ophthalmic infection, use 2 g/day until improving.
- conjunctivitis (child)
  - ceftriaxone 50 mg/kg (max 125 mg) i.m. once
  - if deep ophthalmic infection use 50–100 mg/kg/day until improving.
- HIV-positive patients – no change to the above treatment.

Sexual contacts

In most cases, patients should be referred to GU medicine specialists for management. Health advisers will make arrangements to screen and treat sexual partners. Patients should be advised to avoid unprotected sexual intercourse until they and their partner(s) have completed treatment and follow-up.

Discuss ways of reducing the risk of acquiring STIs in the future, i.e. reducing the number of partners and using condoms.

Other management

About one-fifth of people with gonorrhoea also have a genital *Chlamydia trachomatis* infection. Patients should therefore be tested for this and should be advised to take epidemiological treatment (see page 95). Patients should be advised to have a check up for other STIs including HIV.

The need for a test of cure (TOC) is debatable. If symptoms have resolved from the affected areas and an antibiotic was used to which the organism was sensitive then a TOC is probably not needed.

If the patient was culture positive from a site at which they were asymptomatic then there is still value in doing a TOC. This is particularly true of pharyngeal infection where treatment failure is more common. A TOC is best done at around 10–14 days following treatment and gives an opportunity to review treatment of contacts. The specimens for the TOC should be taken from all sites where the infection was initially diagnosed. If the pharynx was not swabbed at initial presentation, it should be swabbed now because infection can be harder to eradicate from this site.

If gonorrhoea is diagnosed in a child, consider sexual abuse and discuss with a consultant community paediatrician.

Consider an ophthalmology referral for someone (adult or child) with gonococcal conjunctivitis, since corneal ulceration and further ocular damage can occur rapidly.

Further reading

Bignell C. UK National guideline on management of gonorrhoea in adults.
  http://www.bashh.org/guidelines/gc%200601.pdf

Hepatitis B infection

Gordon McKenna

Introduction and epidemiology

Hepatitis B is a DNA virus with particular affinity for replicating within hepatic tissue. It is the most infectious virus likely to be met in common clinical practice, with significant morbidity and mortality on a global basis. The likelihood of transmission is dependent on virus infectivity, viral load and host factors, particularly underlying immunity. It is most likely to be spread by the parenteral route, but sexual activity and close social contact are also important mechanisms. Mother-to-child transmission, particularly during parturition and breast feeding, are well recognized. A recent study estimated that about 18% of acute hepatitis B infections in the UK were from sexual transmission. In countries of medium or higher prevalence, this figure is likely to be higher.

Hepatitis B is a notifiable infection. In 2001, 549 cases were notified to the Health Protection Agency in England and Wales. The national incidence rate has been reasonably constant over time, with sporadic outbreaks occurring in at-risk groups.

The prevalence of hepatitis B in the population varies with the recognized risk factors for the infection. The background prevalence in the general UK population of antibodies to hepatitis B core antigen (antiHBc) is around 0.1%. In persons with a history of injecting drug use, antiHBc, the marker for past exposure, was in 2001 present in 21% of males who had injected in the previous 3 years. In a study of attendees of a London GUM clinic published in 1998, past exposure of 38.7% was noted in men having sex with men, and 5.9% in heterosexual men.

On a national basis, London tends to have a higher prevalence of hepatitis B than the rest of England, and Scotland has a lower prevalence than England.

Globally, South East Asia has a high prevalence of hepatitis B, with figures of circa 5% of chronic carriage in the general population. Some interesting cultural differences exist within many countries; e.g. Maori have a much higher prevalence than non-Maori in New Zealand.

Presentation

It is well recognized that any patient with abnormal liver function tests or jaundice should be screened for the common hepatitis viruses, irrespective of the presence of risk factors. Other common causes of hepatitis are alcohol, Epstein Barr and cytomegalovirus, or medication. Recent travel to an overseas country is an important risk factor of hepatitis, particularly hepatitis A, E and G.

Subclinical infections with hepatitis B are well recognized. This may manifest as a patient with no past history of jaundice who is subsequently shown to be positive for antiHBc antibodies, indicating past exposure. Patients may also present with circulating hepatitis B surface antigen (HBsAg), usually indicating chronic carriage of hepatitis B. The persistence of surface antigen after an acute infection is much commoner if the infection is acquired as a child and particularly as a neonate, when rates of 50% are possible. An adult acquiring the infection is much less likely to become a chronic carrier (7%). Hepatitis B infection also has important extra-hepatic features: vasculitis, glomerulonephritis, arthritis and the dermatological condition livedo reticularis.

Complications

If hepatitis B persists for more than 6 months, it is regarded as a chronic infection. After that point, less than 1% of patients per year spontaneously seroconvert and clear circulating antigen.

Chronic carriage is likely to lead to the serious sequelae of chronic hepatitis: cirrhosis and portal hypertension in around 20%. It is estimated that 350 million people globally have chronic hepatitis B, with 1–2 million deaths each year from its complications. It is likely that hepatocellular carcinoma represents the single biggest preventable cancer (by vaccination) in the world. The development of features of hepatocellular carcinoma on top of the ill-health of chronic hepatitis B can be subtle in the early stages. A history of weight loss, enlarging liver and rising alpha-fetoprotein levels are ominous findings.

All patients with hepatitis B infection should be counselled about alcohol intake and hepatotoxic medication. Vaccination against hepatitis A infection is recommended by some authorities

Diagnosis

The diagnosis of hepatitis B should be considered for any patient with jaundice and/ or deranged liver function tests. There are five commonly used tests for hepatitis B, and their pattern will inform the clinician as to acute infection, chronic (longer than 6 months) infection, past exposure, infectivity, immunity and superinfection with delta virus (hepatitis D).

> Antibodies to Hepatitis B core antigen (antiHBc) indicate past exposure with or without current infection.
>
> Hepatitis B surface antigen (HBsAg) reveals current infection. If positive, it indicates active infection.
>
> Antibodies to Hepatitis B surface antigen (antiHbs) constitute a marker of immunity, either through past contact (in which case the antiHBc will also be positive) or as a result of vaccination, in which case antiHBc will be negative.
>
> Hepatatis B e antigen (HBeAg) is a marker of active virus replication and infectivity (high). The presence of HBeAg increases the likelihood of transmission tenfold.
>
> The presence of antibodies to hepatitis B e antigen (antiHBe) makes transmission much less likely.
>
> Hepatitis D infection (delta infection) is a superinfection with another hepatic virus than can only replicate in the presence of hepatitis B. It is often associated with fulminant hepatitis.

Specialized laboratories can also test for hepatitis B DNA, hepatitis B viral load and hepatitis B gene sequencing; the latter is useful in typing viral strains.

Treatment

Acute infection

General measures include supportive therapy for mild infections. Once the diagnosis is confirmed, contact tracing is mandatory as it is a notifiable infection. Vaccination of close family and sexual partners is recommended.

For more severe infections, admission to a specialist unit is recommended. Fulminant hepatic failure occurs in 1% of all cases. In cases unresponsive to all medical measures, liver transplantation may be life-saving .

Chronic infection
General

Apply supportive measures. Advise alcohol abstinence. Advise that the infection is sexually transmissible if HBsAg, HBeAg or DNA is positive and that condoms should be used or abstinence should be practised.

Specific treatment

Specialist opinion is recommended. The use of interferon-alpha treatment is now well established, but should be used with caution as it can make the hepatitic process more active in the short term. Specific antiviral treatments, including adefovir, tenofovir and lamivudine are also used.

Other management

Vaccination

Hepatitis B vaccine contains inactivated biosynthetic HBsAg adsorbed on aluminium hydroxide. There are two vaccines for hepatitis B infection: Engerix B (GlaxoSmith-Kline), with 20 IU of antigen, and HBvaxPRO (Aventis Pasteur), with 10 IU. Reduced dose vaccines exist for adolescents and younger children. Accelerated or superaccelerated courses appear to achieve a greater compliance than the standard regimen.

Immunization takes up to 6 months to confer adequate protection, and a booster at 5 years after the primary course may be sufficient to maintain immunity in those at continued risk.

Many countries have adopted a universal vaccination programme, and children are usually vaccinated in the pre-school years. In the United Kingdom, with a low prevalence of hepatitis B, a targeted vaccine campaign to cover at-risk groups exists; vaccination is therefore offered to:

- all close social contacts of someone with acute or chronic active hepatitis B infection
- all sexual contacts of someone with acute or chronic active hepatitis B infection
- all injecting drug users
- haemophiliacs
- health care professionals

- other occupational risk groups, e.g. police, prison wardens, morticians
- inmates of custodial institutions
- travellers to areas of high prevalence who are at increased risk or who plan to remain there.

The clinical effectiveness guidelines of the British Association for Sexual Health and HIV (BASHH) also recommend hepatitis B vaccination to men who have sex with men, sex workers and their clients, and overseas travellers to endemic areas who are likely to have sexual intercourse.

The Royal College of General Practitioners has recommended that all illicit drug users whether smoking, snorting or injecting should be offered the vaccine.

Post-exposure prophylaxis

In cases where there is likely to have been exposure to hepatitis B, e.g. a needlestick injury from an index with hepatitis B, it is recommended that the contact should receive hepatitis B vaccination and receive passive immunization with hepatitis B immunoglobulin. Infants born to mothers who are hepatitis B positive should receive both hepatitis B vaccination and passive immunoglobulin, unless the mother has antibodies to HBeAg (anti-HBeAg antibodies), in which case only vaccination is recommended.

Sexual contacts

Sexual and household contacts of people who are infectious (HBsAg, HBeAg and DNA positive) should be vaccinated. Partner notification should be performed if the index is infectious. Unless there is a clear historic risk event that is thought to have led to acquisition, partner notification should be performed for an indefinite number of partners.

Further reading

Brook M. Sexual transmission of hepatitis A–E and G. Sex Transm Infect 1998;74:395.

Gilson RJC, de Ruiter A, Waite J et al. Hepatitis B infection in patients attending a genitourinary clinic – risk factors and vaccine coverage. Sex Transm Infect 1998;74:110–15.

Hepatitis B. In: Harrison's Principles of Internal Medicine (15th edn). Braunwald E, Fauci A, Hauser SL, Longo DL, Jamieson JL (eds). McGraw-Hill Professional Publishing: New York, 2001.

PHLS Subcommittee. Exposure to hepatitis B virus; guidance on post exposure prophylaxis. Communicable diseases report vol 2. London: Health Protection Agency, 1992. <http://www.hpa.org.uk/cdr/CDRreview/1992/Cdrr0992.pdf>

Zuckerman AJ. More than a third of the world's population has been infected with hepatitis B (letter). BMJ 1999;318:1213.

Herpes

Andrew Leung

Introduction

Genital herpes is one of the most common sexually transmitted diseases and is the most common cause of genital ulcers in developed countries. It is caused by herpes simplex virus types 1 and 2 (HSV-1, HSV-2). The worldwide annual incidence of genital herpes is about 20 million cases. The prevalence of HSV-2 infection is 10–30% in most developed countries.

When HSV is transmitted to the genital mucosa, it starts to replicate within the epidermal cells. This leads to cell lysis, resulting in the formation of vesicles, which then rupture to form ulcers. Not everyone exposed to HSV develops symptomatic genital herpes. A prior HSV-1 infection, usually acquired during childhood, generally protects the individual from later genital HSV-1 infection. Symptoms and signs are also less common if this individual subsequently develops genital HSV-2 infection.

HSV also enters into the sensory nerve endings and moves along the axon to the neurons within the spinal sensory ganglia. It then either replicates within the neurons or enters a state of 'latency'. Latent virus can reactivate either spontaneously or in response to a variety of environmental stimuli, such as ultraviolet irradiation, trauma or stress. It is then conveyed back to the epidermis along the sensory nerves, resulting either in asymptomatic shedding or in clinical recurrences. The frequency of recurrences varies considerably between individuals. In general, the more severe the primary infection, the more frequent the recurrences will be. Many patients with primary genital HSV-1 infection do not experience recurrent infections in the first year; if they do so, the recurrence rate is usually low (on average one per year in the year following diagnosis). However, most patients with primary genital HSV-2 infection have recurrences in the first year and the recurrence rate may be high (on average four recurrences in the first year). For most people, recurrences get less common over time, but about 25% of people with symptomatic HSV-2 continue to have frequent recurrences for many years.

Transmission occurs by close personal contact. This can occur during periods of symptomatic or asymptomatic shedding of the virus. The overall transmission rate for HSV-2 infection to a seronegative partner is estimated to be 5–10% per year. The risk of transmission appears to be highest when clinical lesions are present. However, transmission from asymptomatic partners is more common because the individual with symptoms is likely to abstain from sexual contact, or the partner may not wish to have sexual contact with someone with obvious lesions.

Presentation

First-episode genital herpes
Most infected persons have subclinical infection. When symptoms and signs are present, severity is determined by the presence of prior immunity to HSV. In non-

primary first episodes (patients with prior HSV infection), symptoms are often less severe and resolve more quickly. True primary genital herpes only accounts for about 50% of patients presenting with their first symptomatic episode.

The incubation period is 2–20 days. In most patients, there is a generalized 'flu-like' illness with fever, malaise, headache and myalgia. These systemic symptoms persist for a week and are usually more prominent in women and in those with HSV-2 infection.

Lesions first appear as vesicles and rapidly ulcerate. The number of lesions varies considerably and lesions often coalesce to form a large area devoid of epithelium. Pain is an almost universal complaint. Tender inguinal lymphadenopathy is also common. Without treatment, the lesions remain painful for 10–12 days, with resolution after 2–3 weeks.

The urethra is commonly involved. Men may present with symptoms of urethritis, whereas women often complain of internal as well as external dysuria. Vaginal discharge also affects some women and occasionally uterine and adnexal tenderness is present, suggesting upper genital tract involvement. Rarely, the cervix is involved and appears ulcerated or necrotic.

The perianal area is frequently involved, especially in women. This involvement does not necessarily indicate that the person has had receptive anal intercourse. Lesions in the anal canal may give rise to symptoms of proctitis, including severe anal pain, tenesmus, constipation and rectal discharge. Clinical features of pharyngeal infection, usually after orogenital contacts, vary from mild erythema to ulcerated pharyngitis with tender cervical lymphadenopathy.

Some patients develop extragenital lesions. The most common sites are the buttocks and the thighs. Less commonly, the fingers and the eyes are involved. These lesions can be caused by autoinoculation or in the case of the buttocks, reflect the overlap between genital and buttock sacral innervation.

Recurrent genital herpes

In recurrent disease, systemic symptoms are uncommon and the duration and severity of symptoms are much less. The lesions are fewer, usually unilateral, and normally resolve within 10 days. Complications are rare. About 50% of patients notice prodromal symptoms 1–2 days prior to appearance of genital lesions. These symptoms include genital itching and burning. Numbness and tingling in the buttocks or thighs may also occur. Some patients may experience prodromal symptoms that are not followed by lesion formation.

Complications

Complications of genital herpes occur more frequently in women. The most common complications of genital herpes are bacterial and fungal superinfections and neurological involvement. Symptoms of meningeal involvement with photophobia and neck stiffness may be present in some patients. Less common complications include sacral autonomic radiculopathy resulting in urinary retention, perineal and buttock paraesthesias, and in men, transient erectile dysfunction.

Although rare, neonatal infection can cause severe encephalitis and death. Neonatal infection is more common if the mother acquired the infection in the third trimester, since there would not be enough time to pass on immunoglobulin G (IgG) transplacentally. An obstetrician should be consulted if a woman develops new genital ulcers in the third trimester. If it is confirmed as being a first episode, then the delivery will usually be performed under i.v. acyclovir cover and/or by Caesarian section.

Diagnosis

See page 40 for the differential diagnosis of genital ulceration.

The diagnosis of primary genital herpes can often be made on clinical grounds. Typical appearance of multiple and painful vesicles or ulcers is sufficient to make the diagnosis. In non-primary first-episode herpes and in recurrent genital herpes, diagnosis can sometimes be difficult, especially when manifestations are atypical. For example, genital skin fissures may occur with minor trauma or candida vaginitis, as well as with genital herpes.

Clinical diagnosis of genital herpes should always be confirmed by laboratory methods. Laboratory confirmation will also allow distinction between HSV-1 and HSV-2, which carry different prognoses. When genital lesions are present, HSV isolation is the main method used. The specimen is collected by de-roofing a vesicular lesion with a sterile needle and scraping the base of the lesion with a swab. Where lesions are already ulcerated, the specimen is collected by swabbing the base of the ulcer. This is then placed in a viral transport medium. Specimens that cannot be processed immediately should be refrigerated at 4°C. After inoculation, the cell culture is inspected for the characteristic cytopathic effects, which usually appear within 12–48 hours. HSV is then confirmed with specific monoclonal antibodies that will also allow typing of the isolates as HSV-1 or HSV-2. The specificity of viral culture approaches 100% but the sensitivity depends on the stage of the lesion. About 95% of vesicular lesions and 70% of ulcerative lesions will yield HSV, but only 30% of crusted lesions. Hence, a negative culture does not rule out genital herpes.

Diagnostic methods using enzyme immunoassay (EIA) technology for the detection of HSV antigen are available. The main advantage of this technique is the rapid processing time: results can be available within hours. Sensitivity of the antigen detection test varies between kits. The more sensitive ones are comparable to that of culture, and may perform better in late-stage lesions.

Molecular methods using the polymerase chain reaction (PCR) for HSV have been developed more recently. Their main use has been in diagnosing HSV encephalitis and meningitis in adults and neonates, but many laboratories are starting to use them for genital specimens. PCR is more sensitive than culture, although slightly less specific. Research studies have shown that PCR may be useful in determining the frequency of asymptomatic shedding and in the diagnosis of culture-negative lesions. Specimens for PCR can tolerate wider temperature fluctuations during transport than those required for culture, but the technique requires special containment laboratories, appropriate equipment and expert staff.

HSV serology has limited usefulness in diagnosing HSV infection. The newer type-specific serology can be useful for diagnosing asymptomatic infection, determining the risk of transmitting genital HSV-2 to sexual partners, screening pregnant women at risk of HSV transmission to their babies, and for epidemiological studies.

Management

Although antiviral drugs effective against HSV have been available for many years, the clinical management of genital herpes continues to present difficult challenges. Antiviral drugs can stop the replication of the virus but cannot eradicate latent infection. Nevertheless, current management strategies can improve the lives of most individuals diagnosed with genital herpes.

Antiviral drugs

Aciclovir is the most frequently used drug in the treatment of genital herpes. Side effects are uncommon but may include headache, nausea and rash. It is eliminated by the kidney and may require dosage adjustment in patients with renal failure. HSV resistance to aciclovir has been described in immunosuppressed patients but rarely in immunocompetent patients.

Famciclovir and valaciclovir are newer drugs with higher bioavailability and longer intracellular half-life. They appear to offer at least equivalent efficacy to aciclovir, but with more convenient dosages. They both have a similar side effect profile to aciclovir. Patients with aciclovir-resistant HSV will also fail to respond to treatment with famciclovir or valaciclovir and both drugs are more expensive than generic aciclovir.

First-episode genital herpes

Aciclovir 200 mg (400 mg in the immunocompromised) orally five times per day for 5 days is effective in treating first-episode genital herpes. In more severe cases, this can be extended to 10 days. Treatment decreases the duration of local and systemic symptoms, reduces viral shedding from lesions and promotes healing. These effects are most marked if treatment is initiated early in the course of the infection. Hence, treatment should be prescribed at the time of clinical diagnosis (before laboratory confirmation), unless the infection is already almost resolved. Treatment does not alter the natural course of the illness as treated patients are just as likely as untreated patients to develop subsequent recurrences. Intravenous aciclovir is indicated only in the minority of severe cases requiring hospitalization.

Poor drug penetration to the site of virus replication means that topical aciclovir is much less effective and hence not recommended.

Famciclovir 250 mg orally three times per day for 5 days and valaciclovir 500 mg orally twice daily for 5 days are also licensed for use in first-episode genital herpes.

Recurrent genital herpes

Recurrent genital herpes may be treated with a 5-day course of oral aciclovir, famciclovir (125 mg twice daily) or valaciclovir. The efficacy of this treatment depends on prompt initiation of treatment. Patients could therefore be prescribed antivirals in advance of the recurrence, so that treatment is available for the patients to initiate at the first sign of recurrence (or prodrome). Such episodic treatment reduces the duration of virus shedding and persistence of the lesions. However, the benefits are not as dramatic as for treatment of first episodes, often shortening the duration of the symptoms by only a day or so. As most recurrent episodes are mild and brief, many patients choose just to take symptomatic treatment.

Suppression of recurrences

Indications for suppressive treatment include frequent recurrences (>6 per year) and in patients with significant symptoms or psychosexual problems. Suppressive treatment should eliminate or significantly reduce the number of recurrences. There is no evidence that such suppression decreases the likelihood of subsequent recurrences after treatment is discontinued. However, many patients experience a gradual decrease in recurrence rate over time even without treatment. Hence, suppressive treatment is usually stopped after 6–12 months to re-evaluate the need for continuing it.

Suppressive treatment also reduces the frequency of asymptomatic shedding, and a 2004 study indicated that treatment with valaciclovir reduces the risk of transmission to sexual partners as a result.

The recommended dose of aciclovir in suppression is 400 mg twice daily. This may be reduced to 200 mg two or three times daily if recurrences have been completely suppressed by the higher dose. If the patient continues to experience 'breakthrough' recurrences, a more frequent dosing interval of 200 mg four times per day may be tried. Famciclovir 250 mg twice daily and valaciclovir 500 mg daily are also licensed for use in suppression therapy.

Supportive therapy

First-episode genital herpes should be managed with appropriate supportive measures. Measures for symptom control include pain relief (paracetamol and/or topical lidocaine), salt water baths, micturition in water baths and wearing of loose clothing. In more severe cases, admission to hospital and treatment with intravenous fluids and suprapubic catheterization (if retention) may be required. Bacterial or fungal superinfections may require treatment with antibiotics or antifungal agents. Supportive treatment for recurrent genital herpes is similar but because recurrences are generally milder, the need of such measures should be individually considered.

Counselling and education

Genital herpes is one of the first chronic recurring illnesses encountered by young adults. Its diagnosis often causes substantial anxiety in patients. In addition to guilt, some patients experience depression, psychosexual dysfunction, fear of rejection and fear of transmission. Other patients may direct anger to their sexual partners who may be asymptomatic. Counselling with accurate information about genital herpes is therefore important and may minimize the psychosocial and psychosexual complications.

Counselling starts with an accurate description of the natural history of the HSV and its associated clinical syndrome. The concepts of latency and recurrences should be discussed. Patients should also be familiarized with asymptomatic shedding and their fears of transmission should be addressed. In female patients of childbearing age, the management of genital herpes in pregnancy should also be discussed.

Further reading

Barton S, Brown D, Cowan FM et al. 2001 UK national guideline for the management of genital herpes. http://www.bashh.org/guidelines/2002/hsv_0601.pdf

HIV/AIDS

Kimberley Forbes

Introduction

The acquired immunodeficiency syndrome (AIDS) was first described in 1981 in Los Angeles, and over the following few years the cause was identified and named the human immunodeficiency virus (HIV). It is now thought that HIV species evolved from viruses found in non-human primates, the initial interspecies transmission taking place probably in the first half of the 20th century.

Since 1981 physicians have gained considerable experience in treating patients with HIV and AIDS. Almost 20 antiretroviral drugs in four classes have been developed and in the West, deaths from AIDS have fallen significantly since the mid-1990s. Despite the optimism that these advances have brought, HIV is still incurable and the number of people infected continues to increase. The efforts of the many groups working to develop an effective vaccine have so far been fruitless.

In the UK HIV is usually managed by GUM and infectious disease physicians, although GPs are increasingly being encouraged to take a more active role.

Virology and immunology

Lymphocytes are white blood cells integral to the functioning of the immune system. The main role of B-lymphocytes is the production of antibodies against foreign organisms (humoral immunity). T-lymphocytes predominantly deal with cell-mediated immunity and their main functions are exerted using the T-cell receptor. The subtypes of T-lymphocytes are named according to the proteins expressed on their surface. One such subtype expresses a membrane protein which functions as a co-receptor to the T-cell receptor. This protein is called the CD4 antigen.

Although CD4 is found on other cells, including Langerhan's and glial cells, the term 'CD4 cell' is usually taken as meaning a CD4$^+$ lymphocyte. These CD4 cells (also called T helper cells) have several important functions including the activation of B-lymphocytes and macrophages.

HIV-infected CD4$^+$ cells die, although the actual mechanism of death is surprisingly poorly understood. In the early stages of infection, billions of T helper cells are destroyed each day and billions more are made. Ultimately, though, the body cannot keep up the pace and the number of T helper cells declines. This manifests as an increasing chance of acquiring infections with viruses, intracellular bacteria, fungi and protozoa. A variety of cancers, mostly virally mediated, also become more common.

HIV-1 and HIV-2 are part of the retroviridae family. They are RNA viruses and rely on the enzyme reverse transcriptase to incorporate their genetic material into the host genome.

When discussing HIV infection we usually are referring to infection with HIV-1. HIV-2 is associated with lower viral loads and is thought to be less easily transmitted and less pathogenic than HIV-1. It is found mostly in West African countries.

Transmission

HIV is present in blood and other body fluids including semen and vaginal secretions. The risk of transmission varies enormously with the nature of the risk event (see Table 1).

Table 1 Approximate risk of transmission from a person with HIV [modified from British Association for Sexual Health and HIV (BASHH) guideline for the administration of post-exposure prophylaxis following sexual exposure to HIV]

Type of exposure	Estimated risk of HIV transmission per exposure
Blood transfusion (one unit)	90–100%
Receptive anal intercourse	0.1–3.0%
Receptive vaginal intercourse	0.1–0.2%
Insertive vaginal intercourse	0.03–0.09%
Insertive anal intercourse	0.06%
Receptive oral sex (fellatio)	0–0.04%
Needle–stick injury	0.2–0.5%
Sharing injecting equipment	0.67%
Vaginal delivery (no treatment)	5–20%
Breast feeding (no treatment)	10–15%
Vaginal delivery, on treatment with undetectable viral load	<1%
Mucous membrane exposure	0.006–0.5%

NB. no transmissions have been identified following exposure of intact skin to blood, tears, saliva, sweat or urine.

Numerous factors can increase the risk of transmissibility of the virus. In early HIV infection, the viral load can be extremely high (millions of virions per millilitre compared to tens of thousands once someone has had the infection for a year or so). Therefore, the above transmission estimates can be increased by a factor of 10 if the source patient had recently acquired the infection. Of course, they are also less likely to know they are infected.

Most STIs can facilitate transmission of HIV. The main effect is from ulcerating conditions such as herpes, syphilis and chancroid. For example, people who have HSV-2 are twice as likely to transmit or acquire HIV. Other STIs including gonorrhoea, chlamydia and trichomoniasis have also been shown to contribute to transmission, and non-transmissible conditions such as bacterial vaginosis and vaginal candidiasis also appear to be cofactors.

Globally, vaginal intercourse is the main route of HIV transmission. In the UK in 1987 this accounted for only 6% of the total number of HIV diagnoses. This proportion has increased, and in 2003, 65% of newly diagnosed people were thought to have acquired their infection by heterosexual sex (presumed to be largely vaginal sex). About 80% of these people acquired their infection outside the UK, mostly in Africa.

Most UK-acquired infections are in men who have sex with men. In Eastern Europe and parts of South East Asia, the main method of transmission is injecting drug use.

Stages of HIV infection

Signs and symptoms of HIV infection vary according to the degree of immunodeficiency. The stage of HIV infection can be classified using the Centers for Disease Control (CDC) system (see Table 2). This uses clinical conditions associated with HIV and the CD4 cell count. However, it is important to note that many of the conditions that are more common in people with HIV are due to chronic B cell stimulation rather than CD4 depletion.

The World Health Organisation also has a classification system. Their system is designed to be used without the benefit of laboratory data: only clinical markers are used.

Table 2 CDC classification system

CD4 cell count	Clinical category		
	A	B	C
>500 cells/mm^3	A1	B1	C1
200–499 cells/mm^3	A2	B2	C2
<200 cells/mm^3	A3	B3	C3

In Europe, categories C1–3 are AIDS defining. In the US the definition is extended to include categories A3 and B3.

Clinical category A

Most people in CDC category A are asymptomatic and this stage can last for months or years. Indeed, a small proportion of people are long-term non-progressors and never become significantly immunocompromised.

Category A presentations include:
Seroconversion illness (the production of antibodies against HIV). Fever and rash are the commonest symptoms of seroconversion. Other symptoms include joint pain, oral ulceration, weight loss, muscle pain and fatigue. Seroconversion can mimic glandular fever and can give a false-positive monospot test. About 25% of people have an asymptomatic seroconversion. Viral titres in the blood and genital secretions are very high during the seroconversion illness and people are highly infectious. HIV seroconversion should be considered in all people presenting with a glandular-fever-like illness since missing the diagnosis at this stage has serious implications for the further spread of the virus.

Persistent generalized lymphadenopathy.

Clinical category B

Category B includes symptomatic infection in an adult where the condition is thought to be attributed to HIV infection. It includes all symptomatic conditions except those in category C.

Category B presentations include, but are not limited to:

- Constitutional symptoms such as fever > 38.5°C or diarrhoea lasting longer than 1 month.
- Thrombocytopenia. This is thought to be due to reduced production and immune destruction of platelets. It often responds to antiretrovirals.
- Bacillary angiomatosis (also called cat scratch disease) is caused by *Bartonella henselae* and *B. quintana*. Symptoms include fever and a painful rash.
- Shingles (caused by reactivation of varicella zoster) is more common in HIV-positive individuals and is frequently a presentation of previously undiagnosed HIV infection. Atypical presentations such as multidermatomal involvement and a generalized rash over the limbs or trunk may occur.

Infection with *Campylobacter* and *Clostridium difficile* and viral gastroenteritis are common and can occur with any CD4 cell count. Entamoeba and giardia also occur more commonly in HIV, irrespective of cell count. Salmonella occurs with lower CD4 cell counts and recurrent salmonella bacteraemia is category C.

- Sinusitis is common in HIV, particularly with decreasing cell counts. It should be treated for several weeks to prevent recurrence. *Pseudomonas* may also be a pathogen in this condition.
- Oropharyngeal and recurrent vulvovaginal candidiasis.
- Molluscum contagiosum and warts can occur anywhere and become much larger than is usually seen in immunocompetent people. Both conditions respond less well to treatment than usual.
- Seborrhoeic dermatitis and various forms of folliculitis are common.

Oral hairy leucoplakia is commonly seen with a CD4 count below 250 or so. Usually presents as white ridges on the lateral sides of the tongue. It is caused by the Epstein Barr Virus and does not usually need treatment.

Clinical category C

These conditions are AIDS defining and include but are not limited to:

- Kaposi's sarcoma. Caused by human herpes virus 8. Usually first becomes apparent as a spreading purplish spot on the skin, but can involve any part of the body including the gastrointestinal tract and other internal organs.
- Non-Hodgkin's lymphoma.
- Cervical cancer.
- Tuberculosis (TB). In HIV this is usually the result of reactivation of a primary infection. The rate of co-infection varies geographically, being very high in Sub-Saharan Africa. People found to have TB should be offered an HIV test.
- Infection with *Mycobacterium avium* and *Mycobacterium intracellulare* are usually grouped together as Mycobacterium avium complex (MAC). Infection is common in AIDS patients with cell counts less than 100. Any organ may be affected.
- Oesophageal candidiasis. This can present with heartburn and dysphagia.
- Herpes simplex ulceration persisting for more than a month.
- Pneumocystis pneumonia (PCP). This is caused by *Pneumocystis jiroveci* not *P. carinii* as previously thought. PCP usually presents with a dry cough, fever and

progressive breathlessness. The chest X-ray may be normal and CT imaging may be required. The diagnosis is usually made by performing immunofluorescent microscopy on material obtained by bronchoscopy or on induced sputum. Most cases occur in those who have CD4 cell counts of <200 mm^3, so people with a CD4 count below this figure are advised to take prophylactic antibiotics.

- Cerebral toxoplasmosis. This is caused by *Toxoplasma gondii*, which is acquired from undercooked meat or cat faeces. People may present with headache, seizures, hemiparesis or altered mental state. Typical ring-enhancing lesions are seen on CT or MRI. These may be multiple and are seen in the basal ganglia and cortex.
- Chronic intestinal *Cryptosporidium parvum* infection (>1 month). The parasite lives in the gut wall and infection may be primary or reactivation of latent infection. Diarrhoea, abdominal pain and cramps are common.
- Cytomegalovirus (CMV) reactivation. The average CD4 cell count at the time people develop their first episode of CMV disease is below 30. CMV retinitis may be asymptomatic therefore screening is essential. Encephalopathy and pulmonary and neurological manifestations can occur.
- Cryptococcosis. *Cryptococcus neoformans* is a yeast found in soil. Symptoms are associated with a CD4 count less than 100. Initial infection through the lungs can then spread through the bloodstream to any organ. Meningitis is a common presentation. Skin lesions similar to molluscum contagiosum are also seen.
- Progressive multifocal leucoencephalopathy (PML). This is caused by JC virus, which infects the oligodendrocytes. It causes progressive ataxia, paralysis and cognitive impairment. The typical MRI appearance is of diffuse hypodense fluffy lesions which do not enhance with contrast.
- HIV-associated dementia (HAD) is more frequently an AIDS-defining diagnosis in older individuals. In those HIV-positive patients without AIDS, cognitive impairment rises with age.
- Wasting is a common symptom of HIV and can occur at any stage of infection. Technically it refers to loss of 10% of body weight in the absence of an active infection or identifiable cause.

Diagnosis

Many patients come into contact with medical services without a diagnosis being made, and partially because of these missed opportunities, 29% of people with HIV in the UK are unaware that they have the infection. HIV should be considered in anyone who falls into a risk group. A brief risk assessment and tailored pre-test discussion (see page 12) takes little time and testing should be performed more widely.

An 'HIV test' usually involves 3–4 sub-tests, which are usually antibody based. Most people do not develop antibodies until approximately 6 weeks after infection and this 'window period' can be up to 3 months. However, modern 'fourth generation' tests include a test for an HIV antigen; using such a test ~50% of infected patients would get a positive test at a month, ~95% at 2 months and 100% at 3 months. It is therefore essential to know which test your lab uses before discussing test results with a patient. If someone has been given post-exposure prophylaxis following a needle-stick injury or sexual assault, the window period can be as long as 6 months.

False positives are rare but may occur in autoimmune disease and post-immunization. False negatives are usually due to the window period but may occur in agammaglobulinaemia; however, even in this situation a fourth generation test would still be positive.

Other tests

The viral load measured by PCR detects the concentration of HIV present in body fluid (usually blood). This can usually be detected from 48 hours after exposure. It can be of diagnostic use in testing for seroconversion illness when the enzyme-linked immunosorbent assay (ELISA) test may still be negative; however, false-positive results can occur. It is more commonly used in quantifying the burden of virus present in those who are known to have HIV infection and assessing response to treatment.

CD4 and CD8 lymphocyte counts are used to assess the immune function. The rate of decline of CD4 cells (normal range CD4 500–1400 cells/mm^3) correlates with progression of HIV. The percentage of lymphocytes which are CD4 cells is another useful marker. In addition, the ratio of CD4:CD8 cells can give useful information about the stage of the disease. A low ratio implying late disease.

Treatment

Antiretrovirals have been available since the late 1980s, but it was the introduction of new classes of drugs in the late 1990s that has led to significantly prolonged survival. Combination treatment with these agents has been given the catchy although slightly over-optimistic acronym HAART (highly active antiretroviral therapy).

The four main classes of drugs are:
1. nucleoside analogue reverse transcriptase inhibitors (NRTIs)
2. non-nucleoside analogue reverse transcriptase inhibitors (NNRTIs)
3. protease inhibitors (PIs)
4. fusion inhibitors.

Although effective in combination, resistance can rapidly occur if an inadequate regimen is prescribed or if the patient is incompletely adherent to a regimen. Adherence can be difficult; some drugs need repeated doses through the day while others have to be taken either with food or on an empty stomach.

Antiretrovirals have numerous side effects, including metabolic, haematological and gastrointestinal symptoms. Some side effects can be disfiguring, in particular lipoatrophy (the loss of subcutaneous fat from the face and limbs). Because of these side effects and the need for close monitoring, antiretrovirals should only be prescribed under specialist supervision.

There are conflicting views with respect to using HAART during seroconversion illness. The rationale of early treatment is that the immune system may better respond to HIV infection; this has to be balanced with the potential side effects of the drugs.

There is also a public health case for starting early treatment and reducing transmission during a period when viral titres are high. In view of the lack of a consensus, treatment should only be started in primary HIV infection when people have severe symptoms.

> Current recommendations in the UK are to start treatment when the CD4 count is 200–350 cells/ml³. First-line treatment should be with two NRTIs and either a NNRTI or a PI.

Prophylaxis against opportunistic infections includes:

- PCP prophylaxis for those with a CD4 cell count <200 cells/ml. Co-trimoxazole is most commonly used. This also is protective prophylaxis against *Toxoplasma gondii*.
- Cytomegalovirus prophylaxis with valgancyclovir for those who have a CD cell count <50 cells/mm.
- US guidelines recommend prophylaxis against mycobacterium avium intracellulare (MAI) when CD4 cell count <50 cells/mm.

Immunizations

Immunodeficient individuals may not have a good response to vaccination, and in the face of a falling CD4 count, vaccinations should be undertaken soon after diagnosis. Immunoglobulin may be given if protection is required following exposure to some organisms. The HIV viral load may increase following vaccination, although it is unclear if this has any clinical significance.

Apart from MMR, live vaccines should be avoided in all patients with HIV infection, even in those who are asymptomatic; these include BCG, cholera (live oral) and typhoid (live oral).

All HIV-positive individuals should be given pneumococcal, hepatitis B and influenza vaccines. Tetanus and hepatitis A vaccine is recommended for injecting drug user (IDU). Other vaccines may be required for overseas travel such as rabies, meningococcal A and C, and Japanese encephalitis.

Overseas travel for those with HIV

Certain countries completely prohibit the entry of HIV-infected individuals, although this is now uncommon. It is important to check the individual country's legislation. Advice should be given to reduce risk of food- and vector-borne infections. Adequate supplies of drugs should be taken in hand luggage to avoid problems if checked-in luggage goes missing.

Pregnancy

Antenatal screening should be offered to all pregnant women. If a woman is HIV positive, antiretrovirals can be given, the aim being to reduce the viral load to undetectable levels by the time of delivery.

Further reading

British HIV Association, http://www.bhiva.org
AIDS Map, http://www.aidsmap.com

Infertility

David Cahill

Introduction

In the UK, demands on fertility services are likely to increase. Changing sexual lifestyles are leading to increasing incidence of sexually transmitted diseases, some of which contribute to subfertility. In addition, women are delaying childbearing. Since 1975, there has been a doubling in the proportion of births to women age 30 and over in England and Wales. We know that one in six couples require referral for investigation and/or treatment for subfertility. Recent guidelines published by the National Institute for Clinical Excellence (NICE) and further comments by the Secretary of State for Health have made couples more aware of what may be available, although this often leads to falsely high expectations both of fertility treatments and of service provision. Natural human fertility is low compared with most other species. Peak human fertility (the chance of pregnancy per cycle in the most fertile couples) is no higher than 33%. Because of this, it is quite unrealistic for couples to expect (1) a higher chance of pregnancy than this from any fertility treatment, and (2) considerable effort on the part of scientists and clinicians to try to do so.

Normal expectations from attempts at conception

After the onset of regular unprotected intercourse, 90% of fertile couples should become pregnant within the first year. After 2 years, this rises to 95%. Conversely, 5–10% of normal fertile couples take more than a year or two to conceive. Some couples therefore will present with a delay in conceiving purely by chance, as they have low normal fertility rather than subfertility. The usual criterion to define subfertility, and therefore the trigger to initiate investigations, is a delay of more than 1 year. Investigations should establish a diagnosis promptly and identify couples likely to need referral for specialist treatment.

Causes of subfertility

In Table 1, the major causes of subfertility are listed. They include sperm dysfunction, ovulation disorder and fallopian tube damage.

Disorders of sperm function (abnormal motility, survival or mucus penetration) impair the chances of fertilization. A complete absence of sperm in the man's ejaculate due to blockage or failure of production is most unusual (2% of cases referred to specialist fertility clinics).

Women who are not ovulating may have variable cycle lengths, oligomenorrhoea or amenorrhoea. Polycystic ovary syndrome will be present in 90% of women with oligomenorrhoea and 30% of women with amenorrhoea.

Most fallopian tube blockage or damage is due to *Chlamydia trachomatis* (up to 80% in our clinic). Such damage and adhesions (due to previous surgery or

Table 1 The most likely causes of infertility and their relative frequency, noting that up to 15% of couples have more than one cause for their subfertility

Cause	Frequency
Sperm defects or dysfunction	30%
Ovulation failure (amenorrhoea or oligomenorrhoea)	25%
Tubal damage	20%
Unexplained infertility	25%
Endometriosis (causing damage)	5%
Coital failure or infrequency	5%
Cervical mucus defects or dysfunction	3%
Uterine abnormalities (e.g. fibroids or abnormalities of shape)	<1%

endometriosis) involving the tubes or ovaries are found in about 20% of couples referred to fertility clinics.

Endometriosis and cervical mucus disorders are infrequent causes of subfertility. Minor endometriosis, without structural damage or adhesions, may not even cause subfertility.

About 15% of couples will have more than one cause for their subfertility. Because of this, it is important to carry out complete investigations from the outset rather than focussing treatment on an incorrectly presumed, isolated cause. In about 25% of couples, no definite cause will be found, even after complete investigation. These couples are said to have unexplained subfertility.

Other factors that affect fertility

As mentioned, fertility and the likelihood of successful treatment is reduced as the female partner in a couple gets older. This effect is seen even in younger women, when a depleted ovarian reserve will reduce natural fertility and can be predicted by a raised serum follicle stimulating hormone (FSH) level. Older women also have a reduced chance of success if using their own eggs in assisted-conception therapy.

Other factors such as extremes of weight loss or obesity also reduce female fertility. Being overweight reduces the chances of conception and increases the risk of miscarriage.

Smoking, particularly by the woman, has been shown to reduce fertility. The longer a couple are trying to conceive, the greater the likelihood that they will not do so, particularly if trying for more than 3 years. A previous term pregnancy is associated with a better chance of conception, either naturally or following treatment.

History and examination

Couples should be seen together from the outset, and a full medical history taken from both partners. Measurement of body mass index; assessment for any signs of endocrine disorder, particularly polycystic ovarian syndrome; and a pelvic examination should be part of any examination for the woman. Examination of the man is not usually necessary unless indicated by his medical history or if his initial semen analysis result is abnormal. In most couples the initial history and examination will give little indication of the cause of their subfertility and full investigations will be needed.

Investigations

These can be considered as general investigations (justifiable for any couple desiring a pregnancy) and specific investigations (to help establish a particular cause). Full initial investigations are advisable for all couples. Do not make assumptions about the diagnosis – 15% are likely to have more than one abnormality.

Initial investigations for ovulatory disorder need to be undertaken at specific stages of the woman's cycle:

Progesterone: For women with regular cycles, their luteal phase progesterone may be measured 7 days before the expected date of menstruation (and we advise that the patient ring to confirm the date of onset to ensure validity of the sample). For women with irregular length cycles, their luteal phase progesterone may be best measured at 5-day intervals from 7 days before the earliest expected date of menstruation until the time they begin their next period.

FSH and LH: Measurement of FSH and luteinizing hormone (LH) should be undertaken between days 2–5 in women who have periods or, if cycles are very infrequent or absent, a random FSH and LH measurement is acceptable.

TSH: Measurement of thyroid stimulating hormone (TSH) is important, although it is rarely abnormal, especially in women with regular cycles. However, frank or compensated hypothyroidism is readily treated and, if missed, is associated with an increased risk of miscarriage and possible long-term health consequences for any child.

Prolactin: Hyperprolactinaemia is rare in the absence of amenorrhoea.

SHBG: Sex hormone binding globulin (SHBG) is not a routine investigation, but a low SHBG result supports the diagnosis of polycystic ovary syndrome.

Seminal analysis is the primary male investigation, although it is a poor predictor of sperm function. A poor seminal analysis result is insufficient for making a diagnosis of sperm disorder. If the first result shows a low sperm count or complete absence of sperm, it should be repeated preferably 2–3 months later because of the long development cycle for sperm, which can be influenced by various factors, even by a high fever.

The best initial screen for tubal disorder is *Chlamydia trachomatis* serology. If raised (>1:256), the chlamydia antibody titre is associated with a high likelihood of tubal infective damage. High levels of antibodies indicate current or previous tubal infection and both partners should be treated with an appropriate antibiotic, e.g. doxycycline, azithromycin or ofloxacin (see Chlamydia, page 93). Consideration should be given to lower genital tract infection screening in the presence of high levels of IgM antibody in the screen. We do not advocate contact tracing in the presence of abnormal antibody titre alone. Treatment does not correct tubal damage but prevents reactivation if laparoscopy or other pelvic surgery is carried out.

What treatment options are open to couples?

When positive chlamydia serology or hysterosalpingography (HSG) suggest fallopian tube damage, appropriate antibiotic therapy for chlamydia followed by early referral for specialist opinion is indicated. If either HSG or laparoscopy indicate damage, surgical intervention is effective.

Treatment for disorders of ovulation depends on the underlying cause. Polycystic ovary syndrome (PCOS) accounts for most cases of oligomenorrhoea, and about one-third of those with amenorrhoea. A recent consensus document has been published jointly by the European Society for Human Reproduction and Embryology and the American Society for Reproductive Medicine and this provides further details on the diagnostic categories required to fulfil the diagnosis of PCOS. In primary care, more can be done for the treatment of ovulatory dysfunction than for other causes of subfertility. Simple treatments to induce ovulation include clomifene citrate and, for women with hyperprolactinaemia, dopamine agonists. Clomifene citrate (usually given from cycle days 2–6 inclusive) promotes the release of additional FSH and LH to stimulate follicular development. The starting daily dose should not exceed 50 mg and probably should never exceed 100 mg daily in primary care except in very obese women. Mid-luteal serum progesterone measurements can be used to check for an ovulatory response. Follicle numbers could also be monitored by ultrasound, but there is no convincing evidence that this reduces the risk of multiple pregnancy (mainly twins) with clomifene, which is about 8%. Because of a possible association with later borderline ovarian tumours, clomifene should not be prescribed in nulliparous women for more than 12 months.

Dopamine agonists such as bromocriptine and cabergoline are safe and effective treatments for hyperprolactinaemia. However, the diagnosis and monitoring of women with presumed hyperprolactinaemia can be sufficiently complicated to warrant specialist referral. It is worth considering pharmacological causes for hyperprolactinaemia, such as dopamine antagonists, some antihypertensives and major tranquillizers, before referral. It is unlikely that dopamine agonist therapy will overcome an iatrogenic cause of raised prolactin levels.

In the treatment of women with PCOS, there has been recent interest in the use of metformin. It has been shown to increase SHBG, presumed to be a secondary response of reducing hyperinsulinaemia, and thus reduce free testosterone levels in circulation. It also reduces LH concentrations and ovarian sensitivity to LH. Over 90% of women with oligomenorrhoea or amenorrhoea undergoing treatment with metformin have been reported to experience a return of normal cycles, with 20% conceiving within 6 months of treatment.

The starting dose of metformin is 500 mg daily. At this dose, we find that many women get more regular ovulatory cycles. If not, the dose may be increased to 500 mg twice daily for 3 months minimum. If cycles become regular, it is worth continuing for 6 months at this dose. If the woman's cycle remains irregular, the dose can be increased to 500 mg three times daily or 850 mg twice daily. Serum progesterone measurements at 5-day intervals from day 21 will indicate whether normal ovulation is occurring. Ovulation can be expected in about 30–40% of women with metformin alone. For women who are still not having periods and/or ovulatory progesterone levels, additional clomifene may be used as described above. The combination of metformin and clomifene will induce ovulation in about 90% of women with PCOS. Side effects of metformin include mild nausea, diarrhoea and abdominal bloating. These are minimized by the gradual increase in dosage and are almost always transient. No teratogenic effects have been reported from it being taken in early pregnancy (and some have advocated its use); metformin should be stopped when the woman has a positive pregnancy test.

Couples in which the man has sperm dysfunction need early referral for in vitro fertilization (IVF), usually with intracytoplasmic sperm injection (ICSI), the direct injection of a single sperm into each egg. Where access to IVF/ICSI is not possible, there is the option of donor insemination.

For infertile women with endometriosis, clomifene may help optimize fertility if the duration of subfertility is less than 3 years. In the remainder, IVF is the most effective treatment to achieve a pregnancy, and early referral to a specialist clinic is advised.

Provision of IVF and other assisted reproduction therapies will continue to be less than transparent and of variable availability in the UK for some time. All couples who are infertile can expect to have certain levels of service provision, through NICE, such as three cycles of IVF or ICSI treatment. This is likely to occur at different rates in different parts of the UK, while the full implication of the NICE guidelines is considered.

Summary

In this section, the causative and contributory factors for infertility and the management options are reviewed, with a particular emphasis on treatment in primary care rather than in the hospital setting.

Further reading

Balen A, Jacobs H. Infertility in Practice, 2nd edn. Churchill Livingstone: Edinburgh, 2001.
Cahill DJ, Wardle PG. Understanding Infertility. Family Doctor Publications and British Medical Association: Banbury, 2000.
CHILD, the National Infertility Support Network, www.child.org.uk
Polycystic Ovaries Self-Help Group, www.verity-pcos.org.uk

Lymphogranuloma venereum

Steve Baguley

Introduction

Lymphogranuloma venereum (LGV) is an STI caused by the invasive L serovars of *Chlamydia trachomatis*. The STI commonly known as chlamydia is caused by serovars D–K. These serovars are not invasive and so do not cause the symptoms and signs of LGV.

LGV is rare in the West, although since 2003 the number of diagnoses has increased significantly, albeit to low levels (about 30 cases in the UK in 2004). Most of the recent cases in Western Europe have occurred in HIV-positive men who have had anal sex with multiple male partners. LGV is still relatively common in parts of southern and eastern Africa, South East Asia, South America and the Caribbean. Its exact prevalence is hard to measure because it is hard to diagnose, although it is thought to cause about 5% of genital ulcers in India.

Although classed as a cause of 'tropical genital ulcers', ulceration is not a major feature of its symptomatology.

Presentation

The initial lesion of LGV is a shallow ulcer which appears 3–12 days after contact and resolves spontaneously. The ulcer occurs in the infected area, which could be the penis, cervix or rectum. Because it is painless, only a minority of people seek attention in this first stage. Sometimes a urethral or vaginal discharge can occur.

Generally people only present in the second stage when the organism has spread through the lymphatics to the local nodes. After 2–6 weeks the draining nodes (usually the unilateral inguinal and femoral nodes) become inflamed, tender and sometimes necrotic. If inguinal and femoral nodes are enlarged, the inguinal ligament will form a depression between them – this is called the groove sign. If the affected nodes are in the pelvis (for example secondary to rectal or cervical infection) then the patient might have no visible lymphadenopathy. Instead they might present with rectal/pelvic pain, constipation or bloody stools. Constitutional symptoms are common due to haematogenous spread of the organism and the node abscesses. In the UK, most people have presented with anorectal symptoms. It is unclear what proportion of people have asymptomatic carriage of the L serovars.

Without treatment, the lymphadenopathy of the second stage slowly resolves and the affected nodes and lymphatics heal by scarring. In some people the scarring is extensive and, combined with persistent infection, this can result in contraction of tissues and blockage of lymphatics. This can result in distortion and lymphoedema of the genital tissues and anal or vaginal strictures. This third stage of LGV is sometimes called genitoanorectal syndrome. People can present with constipation or signs of proctitis.

Complications

Rectal strictures can cause bowel obstruction. The fibrosis of the third stage of LGV can restrict blood supply and hence necrosis occurs leading to fistula and sinus formation. If this happens in conjunction with proctitis, the presentation can mimic Crohn's disease.

Haematogenous spread can cause hepatitis and arthritis.

Diagnosis

A clinical diagnosis can be made in someone with typical lymphadenopathy, no/minimal ulceration, no obvious source of sepsis in the leg and a sexual contact in an endemic country. An attempt should always be made to confirm the diagnosis.

Unfortunately it can be difficult to confidently diagnose LGV, although recent European outbreaks have been a spur to improve the situation. *C. trachomatis* can be cultured from an affected site such as an ulcer or a bubo, but culture facilities are not widely available. Direct immunofluorescence microscopy is quite widely available and is highly specific if material is obtained from a bubo. Most of the nucleic acid amplification tests (PCR, strand displacement amplification (SDA)) should give a positive result.

Microimmunofluorescence serology is helpful; although the assay specific for *C. trachomatis* is not widely available, a high or rising complement fixation titre can be suggestive of LGV, although such titres can also occur in pelvic inflammatory disease and epididymo-orchitis. Tests to distinguish between the different serovars of chlamydia (restriction endonuclease analysis of the amplified outer membrane protein A gene) are usually only available in national research labs.

Treatment

The standard treatment is a choice of:

- doxycycline 100 mg p.o. b.d. for 21 days, or
- erythromycin 500 mg p.o. q.i.d. for 21 days.

Azithromycin is probably effective; a recent patient in the Netherlands was successfully treated with a single dose of azithromycin 1 g, although using the drug once a week for 3 weeks would be a more cautious regimen.

- Buboes can be aspirated under antibiotic cover, although there is usually little fluid in them.
- Analgesia with NSAIDs is usually necessary.
- Genital disfigurement and rectal strictures will need surgical correction.

Other management

- The patient should be offered a check for other STIs, including other causes of genital ulceration, and HIV. Weekly review is sensible to check progress and re-aspirate buboes if necessary.

- Advise patient about reducing the risk of acquiring STIs in the future and that they have no protective immunity against further episodes of LGV.
- Reactivation of LGV following treatment in people with HIV has been reported.

Sexual contacts

All sexual contacts since 1 month prior to onset of symptoms should be seen and examined. The person should be advised to avoid sex until the lesions of ulceration or lymphadenopathy have completely healed.

Further reading

Mabey D, Peeling RW. Lymphogranuloma venereum. Sex Transm Infect 2002;78(2):90–2.
Mayaud P, McCormick D. UK national guideline on the management of chancroid. 2001. http://www.bashh.org/guidelines/LGV 06 01.pdf

Molluscum contagiosum

Steve Baguley

Introduction

Mollusca contagiosa (MC) are caused by the imaginatively named molluscum contagiosum virus, the sole member of the molluscipoxvirus genus of the poxvirus family.
There are four types of MCV with MCV-1 being the commonest. This fact is only of
interest to virologists and epidemiologists, however, since the type of MCV does not
appear to affect virulence or treatment.

Genital lesions are usually sexually transmitted – the virus is spread by close contact
– but it may be possible to acquire MCV from contaminated towels or clothing. In
2002 there were approximately 10 000 diagnoses of MC at UK GUM clinics and two-
thirds of those diagnoses were in men. This sex difference is probably due to the
relative visibility of male genitalia and because women are more likely to visit their
GP instead.

Presentation

Two to 26 weeks following exposure to the virus, an unknown proportion of people
develop MC. The lesions are normally noticed by the patient as smooth, skin-coloured
or pearlescent bumps with a central dimple. When noticed they are often only a few
millimetres in diameter and the central depression is hard to see. It is unusual for
them to exceed 6 mm in diameter, except in HIV-infected individuals where lesions
of 2 cm in diameter have been reported. If the local skin is damaged due to eczema
or shaving for example, the lesions can spread more readily. It is usual to have at
least several lesions.

When a lesion is squeezed, a white cheesy material is expressed from its core.

The lesions usually resolve spontaneously over several months but can sometimes
persist for years.

The main differential diagnosis is with anogenital warts, although the latter have a
characteristically roughened surface. Other things creating diagnostic confusion
include cutaneous cryptococcosis (particularly if the person has HIV), basal cell carcinoma and a variety of benign skin tumours such as syringomata.

Complications

Apart from the large lesions seen in people with immunosuppression or immunodeficiency, there are no significant physical complications. For most people it is a
benign self-limiting condition. Some people experience psychological distress,
although this is less common than with other STIs such as herpes. Sometimes the
lesions heal with scarring. This is usually because they have become secondarily
infected after being picked.

Diagnosis

MC are usually diagnosed on the basis of their typical appearance. If the diagnosis is in doubt, a lesion can be biopsied and sent for histology or the cheesy core material can be expressed and sent for electron microscopy.

Treatment

Although lesions usually resolve spontaneously, this can take many months and in the meantime the virus could have been transmitted to new sexual contacts. Treatment is therefore for cosmetic reasons and to reduce spread to other people.

The range of treatments marketed for anogenital wart therapy usually work reasonably well for mollusca. The following strategy should be effective and reduce unnecessary follow-up visits.

A few lesions

If large, the lesions can simply be squeezed to enucleate them. The area should then be washed to reduce the chance of local recurrences. Otherwise:

- first line: cryotherapy (e.g. liquid nitrogen spray); freeze for 20 seconds and repeat twice following thaw
- second line: podophyllotoxin 0.5% liquid twice per day for 3 days then a 4-day break before resuming if lesions persist
- third line: imiquimod cream used 3 nights per week.

Many lesions

- first line: podophyllotoxin 0.5% as above
- second line: imiquimod cream used 3 nights per week.

NB – podophyllotoxin and imiquimod should not be used during pregnancy.

Sexual contacts

There is no need to trace sexual contacts. People do not need to use condoms with current partners since their partner will already have been exposed to the virus. People should be advised to avoid sex with new contacts until 3 months after the MC lesions have gone.

> Condoms probably offer little protection against MCV acquisition.

Other management

Because MCV is usually sexually acquired, patients should be offered an STI screen. If the patient shaves their genitals they should be advised to stop temporarily since the shaving nicks can give the virus easier access to the skin and encourage further MC growth.

Further reading

Scott G. UK guideline on the management of molluscum contagiosum.
  http://www.bashh.org/guidelines/c12%2004%2003c.pdf

Non-specific urethritis

Steve Baguley

Introduction

Non-specific urethritis (NSU) is the name given to the situation when a man has an excess of polymorphonuclear leucocytes (PMNLs) in his urethra, but tests for specific infections are negative. What constitutes NSU therefore depends on the definition of an 'excess of PMNLs' and which specific infections you have tested for.

GUM physicians have heated debates about how many PMNLs constitute an 'excess'. The generally accepted figure is that if you are doing Gram-stained microscopy of a smear of material taken from a man's urethra, then ≥5 PMNL per microscope field at ×1000 magnification is abnormal.

If you are doing microscopy on a 'thread' specimen taken from a first-void urine specimen, the cut-off is ≥10 PMNL per microscope field at ×1000 magnification.

Most STI clinics, lets call them type A clinics, just test male urethras for chlamydia and gonorrhoea. If a man has urethritis but those tests are negative, then he has NSU. Other clinics, let's call them type B clinics, also test for mycoplasma and trichomoniasis. Again, a full set of negative tests means that the man has NSU. As you can see, NSU diagnosed at clinic A is a different beast from that diagnosed at clinic B. So what causes urethritis that is not due to chlamydia or gonorrhoea? Numerous conditions are suspected and sometimes proven to be associated with NSU, as shown in Table 1.

Table 1 Possible causes of NSU

	Sexually transmitted infections	*Infections that are probably not sexually transmitted*	*Other conditions*
Approximate proportion of cases of NSU	85%	10%	5%
Condition	Chlamydia or gonorrhoea with a false-negative test, *Mycoplasma genitalium, Ureaplasma urealyticum, Trichomonas vaginalis,* herpes simplex viruses	Adenoviruses, urinary tract infections, *Candida albicans, Neisseria meningitidis,* chronic bacterial prostatitis	Contact urethritis (e.g. from shower gel), foreign bodies, urethral stricture, chronic pelvic pain syndrome (inflammatory)

Due to the uncertain significance of NSU and increased demands on time, some GUM clinics are stopping doing microscopy on asymptomatic men, arguing that those with chlamydia or gonorrhoea will be picked up by the laboratory tests and that there is insufficient evidence of the benefit of treating other causes of urethritis. Further research might clarify the situation – it might reveal that *U. urealyticum*, for example, is definitely associated with a late complication such as infertility and thus screening for it is useful.

Non-gonococcal urethritis (NGU) is a term that is sometimes (incorrectly) used interchangeably with NSU. As the name suggests, NGU is urethritis when the tests for gonorrhoea are negative. About 40% of cases of NGU are due to chlamydia.

NSU and NGU are only diagnosed in men; the equivalent diagnosis in women is non-specific cervicitis, although this diagnosis is rarely made in practice. This is because it is even more difficult to confidently judge what constitutes an excess of PMNLs on a specimen from the cervix.

Presentation

Most men with NSU are asymptomatic and are diagnosed when they present to a GUM clinic looking for an STI screen.

Some men with NSU have symptoms such as dysuria, discharge (usually scanty or clear) or vague feelings of urethral irritation. The men with NSU that GPs encounter are more likely to be in this latter group. Merely having symptoms is not enough to diagnose NSU; in the absence of microscopic evidence of urethritis, dysuria might just be due to urethral irritation (see Dysuria and urethral discharge, page 29).

Complications

These depend on the causative organism or condition, although by definition, in NSU the cause is not known. Possibilities include Reiter's syndrome, epididymo-orchitis and transmission to women leading to premature labour (*T. vaginalis*) or infertility (chlamydia).

Diagnosis

The diagnostic criteria for NSU are described in the introduction. The longer a man holds his urine, the greater the sensitivity of the test. An absolute minimum hold is 1 hour, but a hold of more than 4 hours is better. If microscopy is normal after this delay, a symptomatic man should be asked to return having held his urine overnight. The specimen should be collected using a small tipped swab or a plastic loop. This material should then be smeared over about 0.5 cm^2 of a microscope slide and sent to the lab for microscopy.

Dipstick urinalysis of a first-void urine specimen can sometimes reveal leucocytes, but this is a less sensitive test for urethritis. If the patient has urinary frequency, urgency or haematuria, a midstream specimen of urine should be taken and sent for microscopy, culture and sensitivity.

Chlamydia and gonorrhoea should be excluded.

Treatment

Standard treatments for *Chlamydia trachomatis* are usually effective for NSU. For example:

- azithromycin 1 g p.o. once
- or doxycycline 100 mg p.o. b.d. for 7 days.

Some people have persistent symptoms despite taking treatment correctly and not having sex with untreated partners. The cause of these symptoms is unknown. If urethritis is confirmed by microscopy the patient should be offered second-line treatment with:

- erythromycin 500 mg four times a day for 2 weeks
- and metronidazole 400 mg twice a day for 5 days.

If the patient has a history of flow abnormality or a 'blockage' in the urethra, he could be referred for urological assessment using urethroscopy as a check for a urethral stricture or foreign body.

Sexual contacts

Most causes of NSU are sexually transmitted infections, so the patient's sexual contacts need to be seen. Because there are no useful definitive tests to see if a partner has acquired the causative agent, they should be offered treatment epidemiologically.

If the man is asymptomatic, all sexual contacts within the previous 6 months should be seen. If he is symptomatic, going back 4 weeks prior to the onset of symptoms should be enough. Contacts should have a history taken and be offered treatment with a first-line agent as documented above. They should abstain from sex until both partners have finished treatment.

If symptoms persist in the index case following adequate treatment of the couple, the contact does not need to be retreated.

Further management

Information about NSU should be given. If the NSU is thought to be sexually acquired, the patient should be offered tests for other STIs including HIV.

Further reading

Horner PJ, Shahmanesh M. National guideline on the management of non-gonococcal urethritis. www.bashh.org\guidelines\NGU 09 01c.pdf

Pediculosis pubis (crab lice)

Steve Baguley

Introduction

Rather confusingly, pediculosis pubis is not caused by a louse of the *Pediculosis* genus but by *Phthirus pubis*. It infests parts of the body covered with coarse hair such as the armpits and anogenital region, the latter being the most commonly infested site. The lice can also be found on the beard and moustache and sometimes the eyelids. Infestation of scalp hair is occasionally reported, particularly in those with long hair, although this is unusual. Infestation of the eyebrows and lashes is more common in children.

Phthirus pubis is mostly transmitted by close body contact and that usually means sex. Clearly condoms do not prevent transmission. Non-sexual transmission can also occur, e.g. by sharing a bed, towel or clothing with an infested person.

Once on a new host, the female usually lays two to three eggs per day and 15–50 eggs over her lifetime. The eggs are laid at the base of hairs and hatch within 6–8 days. The eggs and their empty cases (collectively called nits) are the most visible aspect of the infestation. The lice live for about 30 days, maturing from nymphs to adults.

Nymphs and adults do not move around much – they can stay attached and feeding for hours or days on one spot without removing their mouth parts from the skin, sucking blood intermittently. Neither nymphs nor adults can survive more than a day without feeding.

Presentation

The interval from acquisition to the onset of symptoms is usually between 5 days and several weeks. The commonest symptom is itch, particularly of the genital area or armpits. The patient might have seen the lice or nits in the hair or noticed small blue spots caused by bleeding into the skin. Sometimes people notice specks of dried blood in their underwear. The itch is caused by a hypersensitivity reaction to the saliva and faeces of the lice. This reaction can be quite mild and lead to people having persistent asymptomatic infection.

Complications

Unlike body lice, crab lice are not vectors of human diseases. The worst physical complication is secondary infection of excoriations but this is uncommon. Psychological distress is perhaps the most common 'complication'. Parasitic lice arouse feelings of repugnance and many people understandably find the whole experience of seeing insects feeding on their genitals deeply unpleasant.

Diagnosis

This hinges on seeing the lice or nits, the latter being easier to spot as 1-mm-long mid-brown ovoid objects stuck tightly onto the hairs. The lice themselves are 2 mm in diameter, flattened, pale brown, crab-like creatures and often quite scanty.

If needed, the diagnosis can be confirmed using light microscopy. This could be useful if you want to distinguish between head and pubic lice in someone with an infestation somewhere on the head. Head and body lice are noticeably elongated compared to crab lice, although this is usually apparent even to the naked eye.

Treatment

Treatments recommended by the UK National STI Management Guideline include:

- Malathion 0.5% aqueous preparation. Apply to dry hair and wash out after 12 hours, i.e. overnight.
- Permethrin 5% Lyclear dermal cream. Apply to damp hair and wash out after 12 hours.
- These should be applied to all hairy parts of the body plus the moustache/beard.
- Alcoholic versions of these chemicals should not be used as they can exacerbate excoriations.
- Both are safe in pregnancy and breast feeding.

Infestation of eyelashes can be treated with permethrin 1% lotion (keep the eyes closed during the 10-minute application).

Lice can also be removed using forceps or suffocated by applying petroleum jelly.

Insecticides are less effective against eggs than against the lice themselves. The implication of this is that ideally people should be routinely retreated 1 week later. Alternatively, patients could be asked to examine themselves for lice after a week and only re-treated if necessary. If, despite a second course of treatment, the infestation persists try another agent.

Nits can be removed using a nit comb or fingers.

Symptoms can persist for a week or more after successful treatment due to the hypersensitivity reaction – this can be relieved using antihistamines.

Sexual contacts

It is sensible to offer epidemiological treatment to current sexual partners. Patients should be advised to avoid close body contact until they and their sexual partners have completed treatment and follow-up.

Due to the incubation period, sexual contacts in the previous 3 months should be offered an examination.

Other management

- Ideally, patients should be given written information about the condition and its treatment.
- Since crab lice are usually sexually transmitted, it is sensible to offer a full STI screen.
- Consider sexual abuse in children found to have the condition (although it is usually innocently acquired from bed sharing).
- Bedding and clothing might be temporarily infested – it should be washed on a hot cycle, dry-cleaned or sealed in a plastic bag for 2 weeks.

Further reading

Scott G. National guideline on the management of pediculosis pubis.
   http://www.bashh.org/guidelines/pubic%20lice%2009%2001b.pdf

Pelvic inflammatory disease

Steve Baguley

Introduction and epidemiology

Pelvic inflammatory disease (PID) is a common, serious and yet poorly understood condition. It is characterized by inflammation of some or all of the following sites: the endometrium, salpinges (fallopian tubes), ovaries and peritoneum (thus leading to periappendicitis and perihepatitis). However, the term PID is only used if the infection ascended through the cervix.

> Symptoms can vary from non-existent to very severe and it can occasionally be fatal. It is a multifactorial problem – numerous organisms are implicated as causative but the role of host immunity is also important.

The incidence of PID is hard to estimate; the definition varies between countries and even between clinics. Many cases are mild and go unnoticed by the patient or are mistakenly diagnosed as other conditions. When pelvic symptoms occur in conjunction with a confirmed diagnosis of chlamydia or gonorrhoea, it is easier to estimate incidence, although the adoption of more sensitive tests for both infections (see pages 95 and 121) has made modern figures hard to compare with historic data.

The data provided by UK GUM clinics provides some useful clues as to how common PID is. Chlamydia and gonorrhoea are recorded as uncomplicated or complicated cases. Complicated cases include conditions such as reactive arthritis, septic arthritis and disseminated gonorrhoea, but in women the main condition that these figures represent is PID. In 2003 there were 2094 female cases of complicated chlamydia recorded by English GUM clinics, 313 cases of complicated gonorrhoea and 10 736 cases of complicated 'non-specific genital infection'. Of course, these figures do not count the women who were so ill that they were admitted straight to hospital or those who saw their GP, nor does it count those whose symptoms were so mild that they did not seek medical attention.

The age group most likely to have PID is the age group that is most likely to have chlamydia or gonorrhoea, i.e. sexually active teenagers.

Causation

Chlamydia trachomatis and *Neisseria gonorrhoeae* are the two organisms most often implicated in cases of PID, although the proportion of cases caused by each organism varies widely round the world and even around the UK. From the English figures above it can be seen that only 15.9% and 2.4% of complicated cases were caused by chlamydia and gonorrhoea respectively. In the majority of cases (81.7%) no specific diagnosis was made. This is for a number of possible reasons:

- The pelvic infection was due to chlamydia or gonorrhoea and there were organisms on the cervix, but tests done on specimens from cervix were falsely negative. Test sensitivity has improved but even with the best tests 1 in 20 of those with chlamydia will get a falsely negative result.
- The pelvic infection was due to chlamydia or gonorrhoea but no infection was present on the cervix. It is unclear how often this happens but it is theoretically possible.
- The pelvic infection was due to another organism for which tests are not available. A wide variety of other organisms have been implicated including *Mycoplasma hominis* and anaerobes. *M. hominis* can cause salpingitis in experimental situations and has been isolated from women with PID, but the extent of its contribution is unclear. Anaerobes appear to cause secondary infection, involving salpinges chronically infected by chlamydia and sometimes resulting in a tubal abscess. Bacterial vaginosis is associated with PID and most regimens include antibiotics that provide anaerobic cover.
- It was not a pelvic infection at all. The differential diagnosis of pelvic pain is wide including gastrointestinal problems, urinary tract infections, ectopic pregnancy and appendicitis.

What proportion of women who catch chlamydia or gonorrhoea will get PID? Again this is hard to say. Looking at the English GUM clinic data, the complicated chlamydia and gonorrhoea cases represented 4.24% and 4.16% of total female cases of those infections, respectively. Experimental evidence suggests that around 60% of cases of PID are subclinical, so overall a woman stands about a 10% chance of developing a pelvic infection if she acquires chlamydia or gonorrhoea.

Numerous factors can increase or reduce the chance of an ascending infection:

- Exogenous progestogens, e.g. Depo-Provera or the progestogen-only pill, thicken cervical mucus and thus present a barrier to ascending infection.
- Combined oral contraceptives appear to modulate the immune response to chlamydia thus reducing the chance of tubal damage. Although, interestingly, in vitro oestrogens increase the adhesion and growth of *C. trachomatis*.
- Tissue type. Chlamydial PID is more common in women with HLA-A31
- Uterine instrumentation. Procedures including insertion of an intra-uterine contraceptive device/system, termination of pregnancy and hysteroscopy are all associated with an increased risk of PID.

Presentation

The asymptomatic majority will of course not present and will remain undiagnosed. In general, gonorrhoeal PID has a more acute onset than chlamydial PID and is less likely to become chronic. Symptomatic women present with a wide range of complaints of varying severity. These symptoms include:

- Pelvic discomfort or pain (often bilateral) and usually described as a dull ache. Cramping pain is more likely to represent gastrointestinal pathology.
- Deep dyspareunia.
- Fever is uncommon – suggestive of severe PID.
- Symptoms of peritonitis are unusual.

Complications

Early complications include generalized peritonitis, tubal abscess and death. Deaths are very unusual in the West and usually happen as a result of a ruptured tubal abscess.

Late sequelae of PID include subfertility, ectopic pregnancy and chronic pelvic pain. It is unclear what the chances are of a woman with pelvic infection developing one of these complications since the numerous women with subclinical disease who do not have a complication will not be counted. There are a number of factors that affect the chance of sequelae. These include:

- The number of times a woman has PID. In one study, women with one episode of PID were seven times more likely than controls to have tubal factor infertility (TFI), and following two episodes this relative risk increased to 16.2.
- The severity of inflammation. In the same study, women were 5.6 times more likely to have TFI following severe PID than those with mild disease. However, even those with severe PID were still more likely to be fertile than infertile following the infection.
- The age of the woman. Older women were more likely to have TFI than younger women. This might be because of generally reduced fecundity in older women or because they had had previously undiagnosed PID.
- Use of combined oral contraceptives reduced the chance of TFI by a third compared to non-users of contraceptives.

Diagnosis

Most women are diagnosed clinically – very few will get as far as having a laparoscopy, and although laparoscopy is the gold standard test for salpingitis it is less sensitive for milder disease.

A variety of diagnostic criteria for PID are variable. In general, the more precise the criteria are the less sensitive they become. However, one cannot treat every woman for PID so the following clinical diagnostic criteria give a useful guide:

Symptoms:

- pelvic pain/discomfort and/or deep dyspareunia in the absence of urinary symptoms.

Plus examination findings:

- adnexal tenderness on bimanual examination
- and/or cervical motion tenderness.

Plus near-patient tests:

- temperature over 38°C
- not pregnant. Always do a pregnancy test unless the patient has not had vaginal sex for several months. Missing an ectopic pregnancy would be a disaster for the patient and for your future employment
- presence of *N. gonorrhoeae* on Gram-stained smear from cervix
- presence of an excess of polymorphs on Gram-stained smear from cervix. Conversely the absence of polymorphs makes PID unlikely
- mid-stream specimen of urine (MSSU) dipstick urinalysis normal.

Plus laboratory tests:

- positive chlamydia test
- positive gonorrhoea test
- raised white cell count
- raised C reactive protein (CRP).

Treatment

Treatment depends on the severity of the condition and aims to cover the likely organisms: *C. trachomatis, N. gonorrhoeae, M. hominis* and anaerobes. There is debate as to whether every woman needs to have anaerobic or gonorrhoea cover, particularly if her symptoms are mild. However, unless you are experienced in managing PID and know your local STI epidemiology, it is probably best to assume she has all of them.

The following regimens are from the 2005 UK PID management guideline:

For inpatients (i.e. severe symptoms, unable to tolerate oral agents):

- i.v. cefoxitin 2 g t.d.s. for at least 48 hours
- plus i.v. or oral doxycycline 100 mg b.d.

followed by

- oral doxycycline 100 mg b.d.
- plus oral metronidazole 400 mg b.d. for a total of 14 days.

For outpatients:

- i.m. ceftriaxone 250 mg stat

followed by

- oral doxycycline 100 mg b.d. for 14 days
- plus metronidazole 400 mg b.d. for 14 days.

Pregnancy

PID in pregnancy is associated with miscarriage or pre-term labour. Treatment should therefore be parenteral to maximize efficacy, but doxycycline cannot be used. An alternative is erythromycin 50 mg/kg per day given in divided doses every 6 hours.

Sexual contacts

If specific causative organisms are found, e.g. chlamydia or gonorrhoea, then sexual contacts should be treated for those infections. In the common situation in which the woman's microbiology lab tests are all negative, the sexual contacts should be seen, assessed, have an STI screen and be given epidemiological treatment for uncompli- cated chlamydia (see page 95) pending results.

Other management

- Admit if symptoms are severe.
- Unless symptoms are extremely mild, any intra-uterine contraceptive device or system should be removed.
- Patients should be given written information about the condition and advised to not have sex while undergoing treatment and to avoid sex with untreated partners.

Follow-up

Women should be seen again after a few days to ensure that symptoms are resolv- ing. If they are not resolving, consider an alternative diagnosis and/or refer for a pelvic ultrasound scan in case of tubal abscess.

Further follow-up depends on the need for partner notification progress and symptoms.

Further reading

Ross J. UK national guideline on the management of pelvic inflammatory disease. http://www.bashh.org/guidelines/ceguidelines.htm

Priapism

Richard Pearcy

Priapism is a prolonged painful penile erection in the absence of sexual stimulation. There are two main types: low flow (the majority) and high flow. **Low-flow priapism is a UROLOGICAL EMERGENCY** and if left untreated can cause ischaemic necrosis of the penile tissues resulting in erectile dysfunction (ED) or significant shortening. Low-flow priapism is most commonly caused, nowadays, by the pharmacotherapeutic treatment of ED, especially intracavernosal injection therapy, but any ED therapy can cause it. Other causes include sickle cell disease and leukaemia; some cases are idiopathic. High-flow priapism is usually the result of trauma to the perineum (which may be minor) often several days before. The injury results in an abnormal arterial–sinusoidal shunt that causes engorgement of the penis. Table 1 is useful to distinguish between the two types of priapism described.

Table 1 Clinical features of low-flow and high-flow priapism

	Low flow	*High flow*
Rigidity	Firm	Semi-firm
Pain	Yes	No
Duration	Short	May be days
ED treatment	Often	No
Trauma	No	Often
Hyperviscosity	Possible	No

The treatment of priapism is shown in Figure 1 opposite.

Further reading

Martin-Morales A, Rodriguez-Vela L, Meijide F et al. Specific aspects of erectile function in urology/andrology (review). Int J Impot Res 2004;16 Suppl 2:S18–25.

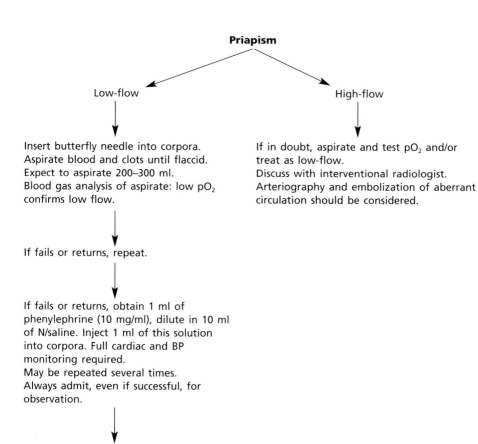

Priapism

Low-flow

Insert butterfly needle into corpora.
Aspirate blood and clots until flaccid.
Expect to aspirate 200–300 ml.
Blood gas analysis of aspirate: low pO_2
confirms low flow.

If fails or returns, repeat.

If fails or returns, obtain 1 ml of
phenylephrine (10 mg/ml), dilute in 10 ml
of N/saline. Inject 1 ml of this solution
into corpora. Full cardiac and BP
monitoring required.
May be repeated several times.
Always admit, even if successful, for
observation.

If fails contact urologist for consideration
of corporal shunt or acute implant.

High-flow

If in doubt, aspirate and test pO_2 and/or
treat as low-flow.
Discuss with interventional radiologist.
Arteriography and embolization of aberrant
circulation should be considered.

Figure 1 The treatments for low-flow and high-flow priapism

Prostatitis

Sunil Kumar and Raj Persad

Prostatitis is an enigmatic condition and has a prevalence of about 5–8% in the USA. It is a condition that has a significant impact on the quality of life of patients. The National Institutes of Health (NIH) has classified this condition into four different categories.

> I – acute bacterial prostatitis
> II – chronic bacterial prostatitis
> III – chronic abacterial prostatitis/chronic pelvic pain syndrome
> IV – asymptomatic inflammatory prostatitis (diagnosed on histology).

Causes

Acute and chronic bacterial prostatitis are infective in origin and the causative organisms are usually Gram-negative uropathogens such as *Escherichia coli*, *Klebsiella* and *Pseudomonas*. Other organisms such as *Enterococcus*, *Chlamydia* and *Mycoplasma* have also been implicated. Patients with chronic abacterial prostatitis present with similar symptoms to chronic bacterial prostatitis but there is no demonstrable infection; in contrast, asymptomatic inflammatory prostatitis shows histological evidence of inflammation in the prostate without symptoms. Autoimmune, chemical and even neurogenic aetiological theories have been put forward for this condition.

Symptoms

Acute bacterial prostatitis is a severe condition with systemic infection; patients present with pyrexia and frequently with severe perineal pain. They may also have symptoms of coexistent urinary tract infection and may occasionally present with acute urinary retention due to prostatic oedema obstructing the bladder outflow tract. Physical examination often reveals an extremely tender prostate with signs of a boggy swelling suggestive of an intraprostatic abscess.

Chronic prostatitis is characterized by a variety of non-specific symptoms such as perineal pain, penile tip pain, lower back or suprapubic discomfort, testicular discomfort, ejaculatory pain and erectile dysfunction. The prostate may be tender or completely unremarkable on palpation and there may be symptomatic overlap with other musculoskeletal conditions that cause pelvic pain syndromes.

Diagnosis and evaluation

The NIH chronic prostatitis symptom index is a questionnaire that is easy and quick to administer and is extremely useful in documenting and following up symptoms of patients with chronic prostatitis. It is also useful in evaluating benefits of treatment and is widely used in clinical trials. Initial midstream urine (MSU) for culture and sensitivity along with blood cultures should be performed in acute prostatitis. Chronic prostatitis is diagnosed using the Mears–Stamey test. This test is also useful in differentiating between the various forms of chronic prostatitis. An initial voided bladder sample (VB1) should be collected, the patient should then void a further 100–200 ml and a MSU sample is collected (VB2). A digital rectal examination along with a vigorous massage of the prostate is then performed. Any discharge from the penis during this time should be collected and sent for culture and sensitivity. This discharge is termed expressed prostatic secretions (EPS). A further urine specimen post-massage should then be collected and sent (VB3).

If the colony count in the VB3 and EPS samples is at least 10 times greater than VB1 and VB2, it is diagnostic of bacterial prostatitis. If VB1 and VB2 show evidence of bacteriuria, then this should first be treated and the test repeated. If the EPS shows <10 polymorphonuclear leucocytes/hpf or if the massage is dry then a count of >10 polymorphonuclear leucocytes/hpf in VB3 when compared with the count in VB1 and VB2 is diagnostic of prostatic inflammation.

Management

Acute prostatitis is treated with general measures such as rehydration, analgesics and anti-inflammatory agents. Broad-spectrum antibiotics should be given orally or parenterally in the initial phase. Oral antibiotics should be ciprofloxacin 500 mg twice daily or levofloxacin 500 mg once daily, and should be given for at least 4 weeks. Complications such as abscess formation should be considered if the patient does not

Table 1 Treatment options for prostatitis

Antibiotics	Quinolones/trimethoprim
α-Blockers	Tamsulosin/terazosin
Prostatic massage	Trigger point release
Anti-inflammatories	NSAIDs
Pain control	Amitryptyline/gabapentin
Biofeedback	Perineal EMG
Phytotherapy	Saw palmetto/pollen extract
α-Reductase inhibitors	Finasteride/dutasteride
Muscle relaxants	Diazepam/baclofen
Surgical devices	TUMT/TUNA/laser
Physical	Massage
Psychotherapy	Meditation/acupuncture
Alternative treatment	Pentosan polysulphate
Heparinoids	Capsaicin/allopurinol
Other medications	TURP/?? radical prostatectomy
Surgery	

EMG, electromyography; TUMT, transurethral microwave thermotherapy of the prostate; TUNA, transurethral needle ablation of the prostate; TURP, transurethral resection of the prostate.

respond to treatment. An abscess, if present, can be drained either transperineally, transrectally or transurethrally.

Chronic prostatitis is extremely difficult to treat and patients should be warned of this problem at the initial stage. Prostatic massage is still carried out nowadays but is of doubtful benefit and has generally been discontinued. Antibiotics even in the presence of a proven infection are sometimes of no benefit in chronic prostatitis. There are, therefore, several other options as listed in Table 1. There are no well-conducted randomized trials showing any benefit in the treatment of chronic prostatitis, hence the plethora of treatments used in this nebulous, poorly understood condition. Alpha blockade is anecdotally reported to provide symptomatic relief by relaxing the smooth muscle fibres in the prostatic stroma and surrounding capsule. Surgical removal is to be avoided unless there are clear indications of potential benefit such as relief of outflow obstruction or the removal of obstructing calculi.

Physical therapies such as heating of the prostate with microwaves have also produced anecdotal improvements

Further reading

Nickel JC. The three As of chronic prostatitis therapy: antibiotics, alpha-blockers and anti-inflammatories. What is the evidence? BJU Int 2004;94(9):1230–3.

Scabies

Steve Baguley

Introduction

Scabies is an infestation by the mite *Sarcoptes scabiei* var *hominis*. Worldwide there are approximately 300 million people diagnosed with the condition each year. In the UK current prevalence is unknown but it is certainly a lot less common than during the Second World War when an estimated 5% of the UK population was infested. The mite is transmitted by skin contact such as sharing a bed and close household contact. It is not easily transmitted by brief touching such as a handshake and is unlikely to be transmitted just by sharing an inanimate object such as a towel. Epidemics occur in nursing homes, schools and other institutions. Although it is sexually transmissible it is unclear what proportion of infections are actually sexually transmitted. Scabies finds itself in this book because for many people, genital symptoms are the most irritating feature of the infestation.

Female and male lice are 0.4 and 0.2 mm in length, respectively. It is usually females that are the colonialists because they are better at gripping skin than the males. When they land on a new host they crawl over the skin (at a rate of up to 2.5 cm per minute) looking for an entry site. A female louse then burrows into the stratum corneum (the top, dead layer of the skin) taking an hour to do so. The female is fertilized by a male which stays on the skin's surface and is therefore more vulnerable to being brushed off. The female lays two to three eggs per day and the larvae crawl onto the skin's surface. The entire lifecycle is about 2 weeks. Sixty percent of mites are found on the hands and wrists but they can also be found in the axillae or under the breasts.

Presentation

During the weeks following acquisition, a new host gradually develops a type 4 (delayed) hypersensitivity reaction to the lice, their eggs and their faeces. This reaction usually takes at least a month to develop but can happen in a few days if the person has previously been infested. Sometimes the hypersensitivity reaction takes a year or so to develop, leading to persistent, asymptomatic infectivity. The main symptom is a generalized itch that is worse at night. Sometimes itching is localized to the genital area or to the hands. On examination of the genitals, one often sees papules and nodules that are a response to the skin being scratched. This is more common in men. Involvement of the head and neck is unusual unless the patient is a young child or immunosuppressed.

Burrows are usually evident in the finger webs and at the wrists as narrow scaly/silvery lines.

Complications

In the malnourished and immunocompromised (whether through drugs, disease or age) the entire body can become covered with burrowing mites. Thick crusts can develop over the palms, soles, elbows and knees. This is called crusted or Norwegian scabies. Despite looking worse, it is usually less itchy than the standard form. Thousands of mites are present on the body and so it is highly infectious. Following excoriation, lesions sometimes become secondarily infected and without treatment, septicaemia can sometimes develop.

Diagnosis

Scabies is usually diagnosed clinically – the patient complains of typical symptoms and the clinician finds burrows in the skin. If you are unfamiliar with scabies or the diagnosis is in doubt for some other reason, other diagnostic methods can be used.

Microscopy
Apply a drop of clear oil to a suspected burrow, scrape some material onto a slide, examine under a ×40 lens to look for the eight-legged mites and their eggs. This is a fairly insensitive test, however, because in non-crusted scabies even a highly symptomatic person may only have 10 or so mites on their entire body.

Burrow demonstration
Draw over them with an alcohol- or water-soluble marker pen, then remove the excess from the skin's surface using an alcohol wipe. The ink enters the burrow and should be visible as a wavy line.

The differential diagnosis of scabies includes, eczema, neurodermatitis and dermatitis herpetiformis.

Treatment

This is aimed at killing the mites and relieving symptoms.

Uncomplicated scabies
Permethrin 5% cream (sold in the UK as Lyclear dermal cream) is the most effective topical scabicide. It should be applied to all the skin below the neck and left on for 12 hours.

Alternatively, malathion 0.5% aqueous lotion (sold as Derbac-M and Quellada–M) may be applied to all the skin below the neck and left on for 24 hours.

Both are safe in pregnancy.

Crusted scabies

- Soak in bath and scrub crusted areas to remove debris.
- Ivermectin 200 µg/kg orally and permethrin may be used as above. The ivermectin can be repeated 1 week later if needed.
- There is not enough data to infer whether ivermectin is safe in pregnancy.
- Sedating antihistamines are useful for nocturnal itch. Crotamiton lotion 10% (trade name Eurax) can be used.

Resistance to most pharmaceutical scabicides is increasing. Tea tree oil appears to be an effective agent which might develop a greater role in the future.

Sexual contacts

It is sensible to offer epidemiological treatment to current sexual partners and close household contacts. Patients should be advised to avoid close body contact until they and their sexual partners have completed treatment and follow-up.

Due to the incubation period, sexual contacts in the 2 months prior to the onset of symptoms should be offered an examination.

Other management

- Ideally patients should be given written information about the condition and its treatment.
- Wash all contaminated bed linen and clothes (ideally >50°C) but if too delicate to wash they can be sealed in bags for a week while the mites die.
- The patient should avoid close body contact until they and their partner(s) have completed treatment.
- Itch can continue for a few weeks even after successful treatment due to persistence of antigenic material in the skin.

Give clear information on applying the treatment – patients must be sure to apply it between the fingers and around the wrists. If the infection is thought to be sexually acquired, the patient should be offered a check for other STIs.

Ask the patient to return at 6 weeks if symptoms persist.

Further reading

Scott G. National guideline on the management of Scabies.
http://www.bashh.org/guidelines/scabies%2009%2001b.pdf

Sexually acquired reactive arthritis (Reiter's syndrome)

Lindsay Robertson

Introduction

A sexually acquired reactive arthritis (SARA) is a sterile inflammatory synovitis that occurs following a sexually transmitted disease. Reactive arthritis can also occur following certain enteric infections but these will not be discussed in detail here.

Presentation

Typically 1–4 weeks following infection, acute inflammatory arthritis will occur. The arthritis is commonly either mono- or oligo-articular (oligo = affecting <5 joints), affects the larger joints (e.g. knee, ankle and wrist) and is asymmetrical. However, fingers and toes can be affected with a dactylitis (inflammation of a digit), where the whole finger or toe becomes swollen and inflamed (sausage finger/toe) rather than

Table 1 Extra-articular features of SARA

System	*Manifestation*
Constitutional	Weight loss
	Low-grade fever
Genitourinary	Infectious urethritis
	Sterile urethritis
	Prostatitis
	Salpingitis
	Haemorrhagic cystitis
Mucocutaneous	Circinate balanitis
	Keratoderma blenorrhagica
	Painless oral ulcers
Ocular	Sterile conjunctivitis
	Anterior uveitis (usually HLA B27 +ve)
Cardiac (rare in acute disease)	Heart block
	Aortic regurgitation
	Aortitis
	Pericarditis
Other	Neuropathy (peripheral or cranial)
	Thrombophlebitis

Adapted from Meehan (2002)

the individual joints of the digit. As well as arthritis, patients may have symptoms of an enthesitis (inflammation where ligaments and tendons attach to bones). Typical sites for enthesitis include the Achilles tendon insertion, plantar fascia and elbow epicondyles. Extra-articular symptoms can occur and are listed in Table 1.

Reiter's syndrome is a type of reactive arthritis and refers to the classic triad of arthritis, conjunctivits and urethritis. It was initially described as being subsequent to infectious dysentery, but it is now recognized that it can occur following a sexually transmitted infection. Approximately one-third of individuals with a reactive arthritis will have Reiter's syndrome.

Young adults are primarily affected. Reactive arthritis secondary to enteric infections affects both sexes equally, but SARA predominantly affects males.

Differential diagnosis

The main differential diagnoses are listed in Table 2. An acute monoarthritis is a septic arthritis until proven otherwise; therefore, joint aspiration, Gram stain and culture of the synovial fluid is mandatory. A chronic arthritis such as psoriatic, rheumatoid arthritis or ankylosing spondylitis can only be diagnosed if the arthritis has been persistent for 12 weeks or more. Therefore, in the acute phase of an arthritis these conditions cannot be diagnosed with certainty but it should be born in mind that an arthritis presenting acutely may be the beginning of a chronic rheumatic disease. In Behçet's syndrome the orogenital ulceration is painful. Reactive arthritis must also be considered as a possible complication of hepatitis B and C and HIV infection.

Pathophysiology

The most common sexually transmitted infection causing SARA is *Chlamydia trachomatis*. *Neisseria gonorrhoeae* (NB, this organism can cause a true septic arthritis too), *Ureaplasma urealyticum*, hepatitis B and C, and HIV are also known

Table 2 Differential diagnosis of SARA

Acute arthritis	Septic arthritis
	Gonococcal arthritis
	Gout/pseudogout
	Rheumatic fever
	Lyme disease
	Hepatitis B or C
	HIV
Chronic arthritis	Psoriatic arthritis
	Inflammatory bowel disease-related arthritis
	Ankylosing spondylitis
	Behçet's syndrome
	Rheumatoid arthritis

Adapted from Meehan (2002)

causative agents. *Mycoplasma hominis* and *M. genitalium* are known sources of non-gonococcal urethritis and may also be causative agents of reactive arthritis.

Active infection with *C. trachomatis* may be asymptomatic, especially in women; therefore, the possibility of a SARA should be considered in an individual presenting with an acute case of arthritis even if there are no urogenital symptoms.

Reactive arthritis occurs in a genetically predisposed individual. Class I human leucocyte antigen (HLA) molecules may have crucial roles with respect to this and HLA-B27 has been particularly implicated. The role of HLA-B27 in the pathogenesis of reactive arthritis is not completely understood. Potential theories include that the infecting micro-organism triggers an immune response by CD8-positive T cells from the generation of bacterial antigens in antigen-presenting cells that are HLA-B27 positive. Alternatively, there may be induction of autoreactivity to autoantigens because of molecular mimicry between antigens from the infecting micro-organism and host tissues. Endogenous HLA-B27 could be the cross-reacting autoantigen and its continued presence would therefore result in the persistence of the inflammatory response. Finally HLA-B27 may act in the thymus to select T cell receptors expressed by CD8-positive cells that react to the micro-organism in a pathogenic manner. These theories are not mutually exclusive, and as not all patients with reactive arthritis are HLA-B27 positive, other mechanisms and/or HLA molecules may be involved.

Investigations

There is no diagnostic investigation for SARA. The diagnosis is clinical, based on the history and examination and is supported by test results. As already mentioned, an acute arthritis is treated as septic until proven otherwise. Crystal arthritis is also an important differential diagnosis. Therefore, joint aspiration for Gram stain, culture and polarized microscopy are important investigations to arrange. Other suggested investigations are shown in Table 3. HLA-B27 is less helpful, because a significant proportion of patients with SARA will be negative. The majority of SARA cases can be diagnosed without performing a B27 test. It may have some prognostic use as its presence correlates with disease severity and chronicity but it is not recommended as a routine test for all patients with suspected SARA.

Treatment

Rest the affected joint(s) with use of heat or ice packs as required. Treat with a full dose of a non-steroidal anti-inflammatory drug regularly. Use supplemental analgesia if required. Intra-articular steroid injections may be required if response to the above is only partial.

Use antibiotic treatment for the infectious disease if still demonstrated to be present. There is some evidence that prolonged courses (i.e. 3 months) may be beneficial for chlamydia-triggered reactive arthritis; however, this is not yet regarded as standard treatment

Extra-articular symptoms are usually self-limiting; however, symptoms of uveitis require urgent ophthalmological assessment. Topical steroids can be used for keratoderma blenorrhagica.

Table 3 Investigations for suspected SARA

Investigation	Results consistent with reactive arthritis
ESR, plasma viscosity, CRP	Elevated
Full blood count	Anaemia, leucocytosis, thrombocytosis
Liver function tests	Elevated transaminases (if hepatitis)
Synovial fluid analysis	Gram stain findings negative, no crystals
Urinalysis	Pyuria +/– bacteria
Cultures	
Blood	Negative
Synovial fluid	Negative

Other useful investigations
Genital chlamydia tests (swab or urine)
Stool m, c and s (to rule out enteric causes of reactive arthritis)
Throat c and s (to rule out other causes of reactive arthritis)
Hepatitis B and C serology
HIV serology (if risk factors present)
Chlamydia trachomatis serology (high titre supports diagnosis although tests not widely available)

Adapted from Meehan (2002).
CRP, c reactive protein; ESR, erythrocyte sedimentation rate.

Prognosis

The majority of patients settle within 3 to 6 months. A small proportion will go on to develop more chronic disease with relapsing/remitting symptoms. These individuals are more likely to be HLA-B27 positive and can also develop sacroiliitis and spondylitis. Due to chronic synovitis in joints they are at risk for joint damage and treatment with disease-modifying anti-rheumatic drugs (DMARDs) is warranted to prevent or slow joint destruction. The first line DMARD of choice is sulphasalazine 2–3 g daily.

Further reading

Lipsky PE. Reactive arthritis and Reiter's syndrome: etiology and pathogenesis. In: Rheumatology, 2nd edn. Dieppe PA, Kippel HA (eds). St Louis: Mosby International: 1998: pp 6.12.1–12.8.

Meehan RT. Reiter's syndrome and reactive arthritis. In: Rheumatology Secrets, 2nd edn. West S (ed). Philadelphia: Hanley and Belfus: 2002; pp 269–75.

Syphilis

Steve Baguley

Introduction

Syphilis is caused by the spirochete bacterium *Treponema pallidum pallidum*. Its genome is almost identical to those of the treponemes causing yaws (*T. pallidum pertenue*), pinta (*T. carateum*) and endemic syphilis (*T. pallidum endemicum*). These three conditions are not sexually transmitted but they are worthy of mention here because of the diagnostic confusion they can sometimes cause (see below).

Syphilis is usually transmitted by sexual contact but it can also be acquired transplacentally, perinatally and parenterally, e.g. by contaminated blood. In recent years a striking proportion of cases in men who have sex with men (20–40%) appear to have been acquired by fellatio alone. There are case reports of other modes of non-sexual transmission, e.g. from bites, but this is uncommon.

Until the mid-1990s, syphilis had been in steady decline in the UK. The infection had become so rare in the US that in 1998 the Centers for Disease Control set up a syphilis eradication program with the headline target of ridding the country of the infection by 2005. Unfortunately the decline did not continue, and since 2000 there has been an increase in the number of cases diagnosed in the US.

Since 1998 syphilis has returned to the UK, although cases are unevenly distributed throughout the country and population. Most diagnoses are made in London, Glasgow, the South East and the North West of England. Men are more likely to have syphilis than women and men who have sex with men (MSM) are more likely to have it than heterosexuals. It is still a fairly rare condition but it is worth keeping in mind as a differential diagnosis. One disturbing aspect of the epidemiology of syphilis is the high proportion of people who have co-infection with HIV. In London in 2001 54% of MSM with syphilis had HIV.

Presentation

'Know syphilis in all its manifestations and relations, and all other things clinical will be added unto you.' This oft-repeated aphorism of Sir William Osler is perhaps an exaggeration, but it gets the idea over quite nicely that syphilis can cause virtually any symptom and sign. It might help to relate the myriad symptoms if you remember that the underlying disease mechanism is vasculitis. For brevity's sake only the most likely or important modes of presentation will be covered here.

Syphilis is categorized in various ways, most commonly into primary, secondary, early latent, late latent and tertiary stages according to the symptoms experienced. It can also be called early or late with the threshold being 2 years in the UK but 1 year in the US. Another distinction is between infectious and non-infectious syphilis.

'Infectious' usually refers to primary or secondary syphilis versus other stages, but this is potentially confusing for two reasons. Firstly, during early latent syphilis intermittent mucosal ulceration can lead to transmission and secondly, syphilis has been transmitted to a fetus up to 8 years after acquisition.

When a fetus acquires this infection possible outcomes include miscarriage, stillbirth and congenital syphilis. Congenital syphilis is also divided into early and late stages although a detailed discussion of its features is outwith the scope of this book.

Primary syphilis

The main feature of primary syphilis is the chancre. A pinkish red macule appears 9–90 days after inoculation. This becomes papular and then ulcerates. Classically the ulcer is solitary, painless and indurated. Sometimes more than one chancre appears and they can be tender if secondarily infected. The ulcers usually last for 1–3 weeks; longer than most cases of herpes, so persistent ulcers should raise suspicion of syphilis. Another distinguishing feature of syphilis versus herpes is that the regional lymphadenopathy that occurs with syphilis is usually non-tender. Dual infections (e.g. syphilis and herpes or chancroid) can occur and cause problems with diagnosis.

Secondary syphilis

In the secondary stage of syphilis the treponemes spread haematogenously causing a multitude of symptoms or sometimes none at all. Rash is the commonest symptom with about 75% of people having one at some point over the following 2 years. The rash is usually reddish brown and macular and can cover all the body, including the palms and soles. It is not usually itchy. In moist areas such as the perineum and armpits the rash can take on a fleshy papular form called condylomata lata.

About a third of people will develop mucosal ulceration that affects the mouth and genitals. This is more likely to be confused with herpes than is the primary chancre, since the ulcers are smaller and multiple. The ulcers and moist papules are infectious sexually and through contact with someone's broken skin.

Other less common symptoms and signs include generalized lymphadenopathy; patchy alopecia; fever; hepatitis and CNS manifestations including meningism, cranial nerve palsies and uveitis. Symptoms can be intermittent over the 2 years following acquisition.

Early latent syphilis

In the UK this is defined as syphilis acquired less than 2 years previously but with no clinical features of the infection.

Late latent syphilis

Many people fall into this category. In the UK it is defined as syphilis acquired more than 2 years previously but with no clinical features of the infection.

It is the usual diagnosis for people with syphilis of unknown duration who have no symptoms or signs. It is important to try to distinguish between true late latent syphilis and congenital syphilis. The history and examination might help with this but not everyone with congenital syphilis has obvious signs. If in doubt consult an experienced genitourinary physician.

Tertiary syphilis

This is very rare in the UK now. Historically 25–40% of people with untreated syphilis would go on and develop tertiary syphilis, which consists of three pathologies: gummatous syphilis, cardiovascular syphilis and neurosyphilis. Symptoms develop 2–30 years after initial infection. It is unclear what proportion of people infected in post-industrial nations today would go on to get tertiary syphilis if left untreated. In the West, treponemicidal antibiotics (penicillins, cephalosporins, tetracyclines and macrolides) are widely used for other indications and it is likely that during the decades of asymptomatic infection a person will take these drugs and either kill the spirochetes or suppress the infection so that tertiary complications are made less likely. If you would like more information about the features of tertiary syphilis, see Further reading.

Complications

Any of the more severe symptoms of syphilis could be regarded as complications. This would include neurological involvement at any stage and cardiovascular syphilis. Foetal infection is almost universal if the mother has primary or secondary infection, but it is unusual in the late latent stage. This can result in stillbirth or congenital syphilis which causes numerous signs including organomegaly, skeletal deformity, anaemia and a wide variety of rashes. Due to the UK antenatal screening program, congenital syphilis is extremely rare with only about 30 cases per year. Most cases occur in women who have not been screened. With the recent rise in the incidence of syphilis, more cases of congenital syphilis will occur, including children born to women who acquired syphilis in pregnancy but after their screening serology.

Diagnosis

Most people are diagnosed using serological analysis of a blood specimen. A wide variety of assays are used but can be divided into treponemal tests (detect antibodies to treponemes) and non-treponemal tests (detect antibodies to cardiolipin). The former almost always stay positive, even after treatment, whereas the latter usually become negative after successful treatment (see Figure 1).

Different labs use different tests, but popular ones are the IgG and IgM enzyme immunoassays, which are treponemal tests, and the rapid plasma reagin (RPR), which is non-treponemal. Other treponemal tests include the treponema pallidum particle agglutination assay (TPPA), the treponema pallidum haemgglutination assay (TPHA) and the fluorescent treponemal antibody (FTA) tests. The only other non-treponemal test in common usage is the Venereal Diseases Research Laboratory test (VDRL). Tests become positive from about 2 weeks after acquisition [the IgM enzyme immunoassay (EIA) usually being the first to react], although it is sensible to allow a window of 3 months in case of delayed seroconversion. Positive non-

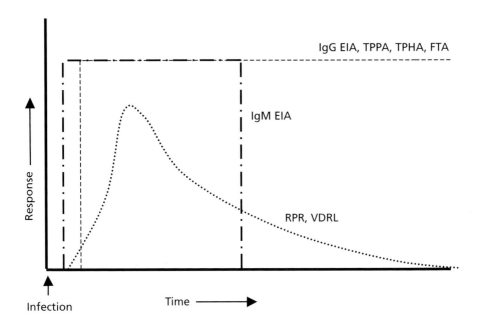

Figure 1 Schematic diagram of the response of various serological assays in untreated syphilis

treponemal tests are presented as titres (neat, 1:2, 1:4, 1:8 etc) and treponemal tests are usually presented as positive or negative.

A treponemal test is not specific for *T. pallidum pallidum*. All the serological tests also react if the person has a non-venereal treponeme (see introduction). A youth spent outside Europe could give a clue that this might not be syphilis. Unusual scarring of the shins could suggest yaws.

In the absence of a clear history of an alternative diagnosis, treat for syphilis. If the person does have yaws, pinta or endemic syphilis, they will be cured by the drugs given for syphilis.

Interpreting syphilis serology can be difficult; this is particularly true if trying to determine whether the person has had a satisfactory response to treatment. This depends on the speed of the fall in the RPR titre and can be influenced by the stage of syphilis and whether the patient has had it before. If the person has antibiotics early in the infection it can modify the serological response; HIV-impaired humoral immunity can also lead to an unusual response or no seroconversion at all. A variety of conditions can lead to false-positive results, this is particularly a problem with the RPR and VDRL tests.

In general it is best to discuss positive syphilis serology with an experienced GU physician.

In a patient with an ulcer, more diagnostic options are available. Probably the oldest diagnostic test available is dark-field microscopy, which uses a modified condenser lens to examine a thin film of exudate taken from a chancre or lesion of secondary syphilis. This is also a good test for people with primary syphilis, when serology might still be negative. It cannot be used for examining oral lesions since commensal spirochetes in the mouth can give a false-positive result. Another problem is that the test is only available if you have the patient near a microscope, so in general this means it is limited to GUM clinics.

PCR tests for syphilis are becoming available that allow diagnosis from a swab taken from an ulcer. Some of the tests use multiple primers to test for syphilis, chancroid and herpes from a single swab. If you have a patient with a possibly syphilitic ulcer, ask your lab if the PCR test is available.

Tests using oral fluid and urine are in development and could facilitate screening in the future.

Treatment

The most widely used drug for treating syphilis is penicillin given intramuscularly. The amount used and the length of treatment depends on the stage of syphilis and whether the person has HIV. Unfortunately, the long-acting versions of penicillin that are most convenient to give are not widely available and there is no international consensus on what constitutes adequate treatment.

The following are commonly used regimens in UK GUM clinics and are recommended in the UK National Guidelines on the Management of Syphilis.

> - primary syphilis
>   - benzathine penicillin 2.4 MU (1.8 g) i.m. once
> - secondary (unless neurological symptoms/signs) and early latent syphilis
>   - benzathine penicillin 2.4 MU (1.8 g) i.m. once per week, two doses
> - late latent, gummatous and cardiovascular syphilis
>   - benzathine penicillin 2.4 MU (1.8 g) i.m. once per week, three doses
> - neurosyphilis (including neurological features in early syphilis) and co-infection with HIV
>   - procaine penicillin 2.4 MU i.m. o.d. plus probenecid 500 mg p.o. q.d.s. for 17 days.

The evidence base for using alternative agents is very scanty. Ceftriaxone, doxycycline and azithromycin are probably effective, but they require further evaluation before they can be recommended as first-line agents. There are increasing reports of *T. pallidum* strains being resistant to azithromycin, although resistance to penicillin has not been reported. This does not mean that the treatment will always lead to an adequate serological response, however.

About 4 hours after the start of treatment, an acute febrile episode (called the Jarisch–Herxheimer reaction) can occur. This is particularly likely in early syphilis. It is unpleasant but rarely causes any major problems. In late pregnancy it can result in premature labour, and in neuro/cardiovascular syphilis it might lead to a worsening of symptoms. The symptoms can be partially relieved by pre-dosing with paracetamol. Despite persisting treponemal antibodies, patients should be informed that they are not immune to syphilis and can catch it again.

Pregnancy

Treating in pregnancy requires the same course of penicillin as would be used for the woman if she was not pregnant. Alternative agents should not be used.

If treatment is completed by a month prior to delivery, then it is likely to be successful in preventing congenital syphilis. At the very least, the child will require syphilis serology to be done at birth, 1 month, 3 months and 6 months. Tests should include the IgM EIA.

Sexual contacts

In its early stages, syphilis is highly infectious, including by oral sex. Therefore, all sexual contacts at risk should be traced and tested. Syphilis can only be transmitted sexually for the first 2 years after acquisition; unfortunately, it is often hard to say when those 2 years have passed, particularly in the common situation where someone is found to have positive serology, no symptoms and no prior testing.

Other management

All people diagnosed with syphilis should be offered an HIV test. This is for three reasons:

1. If they have HIV, they will need prolonged treatment.
2. Syphilis increases the risk of acquiring and transmitting HIV by a factor of four.
3. HIV can result in unusual antibody responses that could make it harder to judge an adequate response to treatment.

Patients should also be offered screening for other STIs.

All people treated for syphilis need follow-up to ensure that the RPR titre is falling at an adequate rate. People treated for neurosyphilis need repeated sampling of the CSF for the same purpose. If the RPR starts to rise again it could indicate treatment failure or reinfection.

Duration of follow-up depends on the stage of syphilis treated, the kind of treatment, whether the patient has HIV and the rate of RPR fall. There is an element of subjectivity involved in deciding whether someone has been cured; whether the person has been adherent to the treatment is an important consideration. For this reason injectable agents are likely to remain popular.

Further reading

Goh BT, Van Voorst Vader PC. European guideline for the management of syphilis 2001, pp 14–27, http://www.iusti.org/guidelines.pdf

Testicular torsion

Sunil Kumar and Raj Persad

Torsion is most commonly seen between the ages of 12 and 18 years. Any male who falls into this age group with acute scrotal/testicular pain should be presumed to have testicular torsion until proven otherwise.

Symptoms

- Acute onset of testicular pain which may be associated with nausea and sometimes abdominal discomfort (as visceral pain may be referred to the abdomen in the T10 distribution).
- The patient may give a history of intermittent episodes of acute pain suggestive of testicular torsion that may have resolved spontaneously (there is a role for elective orchidopexy in this group of patients). There may be obvious testicular maldescent or a history of the testis 'disappearing out of the scrotum' or 'riding high' in the scrotum.

Examination

Typically the patient is in agony with severe pain and there may be associated swelling and scrotal oedema depending on the time of presentation. The testis is seen to be pulled up and lying transversely on the ipsilateral side with overlying erythema and oedema. The cremasteric reflex may be abolished. A reactive hydrocoele may have developed. The testis is always acutely tender on palpation and the patient may not let the examining clinician even touch his scrotum because of the tenderness. The vas deferens can normally be palpated among the cord structures and traced down to the testis. In testicular torsion the vas may be felt to be twisted or is felt to disappear among the cord structures. This sign may often be too difficult to elicit, either because of pain or surrounding oedema

Acute scrotal pain – differential diagnosis

1. torsion testis
2. torsion appendix testes – typically characterized by the blue dot sign on the scrotum if seen early. If the patient presents a few hours after the onset of the pain, scrotal oedema usually masks the blue dot sign
3. epididymo-orchitis
4. idiopathic scrotal oedema – usually viral in origin and not as painful/or sometimes pain free
5. tumour – rapidly growing tumours can present acutely with severe pain and may be associated with signs of inflammation or hydrocoele formation
6. trauma

7. hernia
8. varicocoele.

Predisposing factors

'Bell clapper testes' – the testes and epididymis hang freely within the tunica vaginalis and an increase in testicular size during adolescence encourages the testis to twist around its vascular axis leading to torsion.

Rarely torsions can be extravaginal and this usually occurs perinatally and is seen in the newborn as a firm hard scrotal mass. About 20% of these are bilateral.

Treatment

Immediate scrotal exploration should be performed if torsion is suspected. Manual detorsion may be attempted and should be done in a lateral and outward direction. Usually two to three full rotations may be required to detort the testes completely. If this does not relieve the symptoms, immediate surgical exploration is warranted. If torsion is relieved by manual detorsion, then the testis should be fixed urgently as the manual detorsion may not have relieved the ischaemia completely. If the presentation and findings are not classical, further evaluation is indicated.

Colour Doppler ultrasound can be used to assess blood flow and has high sensitivity with about 80% specificity for diagnosing torsion, but 100% sensitivity is obtained only on surgical exploration!

Nuclear imaging is useful but it delays diagnosis and is not readily available in all centres.

Procedure

The operation is performed under a general anaesthetic. Scrotal incision is made and the tunica is opened, as most of these torsions are intravaginal, i.e. within the tunical sac. The spermatic cord containing the vas, lymphatics, veins and vas deferens can be seen to be twisted. The colour of the testis is noted, the cord is untwisted and the testis wrapped in warm saline gauze. If the findings are suggestive of torsion, the contralateral testis is first 'fixed' – orchidopexy. The ipsilateral testis is once again examined for viability and if viable, is also fixed. If the testis appears non-viable then an orchidectomy or testicular excision should be performed, otherwise abscess formation and severe pain will ensue followed by testicular atrophy.

The testis is either fixed with a sub-dartos pouch or a three-point fixation can be performed. Orchidopexy does not guarantee that future torsions will not take place and parents and patients should be warned about this possibility.

Further reading

Bullock N, Sibley GN, Whitaker RH. Essential Urology, second edition. Edinburgh: Churchill Livingstone, 1994.

Lavallee ME, Cash J. Testicular torsion: evaluation and management. Curr Sports Med Rep 2005;4(2):102–4.

Urinary tract infection

Sunil Kumar and Raj Persad

Urinary tract infection (UTI) is defined as bacterial invasion of the urothelium resulting in an inflammatory response. It usually presents with symptoms of frequency, urgency, dysuria and haematuria. The presence of fever and flank pain should raise the possibility of pyelonephritis. A relapsed infection is defined as the presence of persistent or recurrent symptoms in spite of antibiotic therapy without resolution by culture at any time during therapy. Recurrent infections are characterized by UTI following resolution of the initial infection as defined by negative cultures. Recurrence may occur as a result of either re-infection or bacterial persistence within the urinary tract. Re-infection is responsible for over 95% of recurrent UTI in women. UTI can be classified as complicated or uncomplicated. Complicated infections are those that are associated with an underlying abnormality in the urinary tract.

The majority of pathogens are Gram-negative organisms normally present in the bowel flora. In the community, *Escherichia coli* is responsible for over 85% of UTIs in women. Other Gram-negative organisms such as *Klebsiella*, *Proteus* and *Pseudomonas* are less commonly seen. If *Proteus* species have been isolated, it is important to rule out underlying calculus disease. Gram-positive organisms such as *Staphylococcus saprophyticus* and *Enterococcus faecalis* may also cause UTIs. *E. coli* is responsible for only 25% of UTIs in men. It is also necessary to rule out fungal infections in the urinary tract. *Candida albicans* is the most common genitourinary fungal pathogen. *Mycobacterium tuberculosis* is uncommonly seen but needs to be ruled out as a cause, especially in the presence of sterile pyuria.

Bacterial factors

Bacteria normally reach the urinary tract in an ascending manner. The bacteria have developed specific virulence factors that improve their probability of causing infection. The virulence factors are bacterial adhesins that mediate attachment between the bacterial pili and the glycolipids on the epithelial cell surface. They also produce toxins or proteases that damage the cell wall and enhance their ability to survive.

Host factors

Dilute urine, low pH and high osmolality inhibit bacterial growth. Bladder outflow obstruction secondary to prostatic enlargement, vesicoureteric reflux and urethral strictures greatly predispose to the development of UTIs as they usually interfere with urinary flow. The constant flow of urine washes away the non-adherent bacteria and maintains the sterility of urine. Secretory factors such as Tamm–Horsfall protein also play an important role in inhibiting bacterial growth. Vaginal epithelial cells in women with recurrent UTIs were found to be more receptive to virulent *E. coli* strains than were cells from healthy women.

Diagnosis

Diagnosis is made by sending the urine for culture and sensitivity; urine can be sent in three different ways. Suprapubic aspiration is the best method but it is invasive; it is very useful in infants and paraplegics. Urethral catheterization sampling is only performed in women. The midstream urine specimen, which is the commonest, is prone to contamination. A urine dipstick can provide indirect evidence of bacteria by checking for the presence of nitrites and leucocyte esterases. Microscopy will reveal the presence of white cells and red cells and may suggest an underlying UTI. Urine, once collected for culture, should be stored in a refrigerator and should be cultured within 24 hours. A level of 10^5 cfu (colony forming units)/ml suggests a UTI, but 30% of the patients with UTI may have a count ranging between 10^2 and 10^4 cfu/ml. The low colony count may be because of high urine flow rates, dilute urine, current antibiotic treatment or frequent voiding. The technique of collection is very important and should be indicated on the form. More than 10 cfu/ml from suprapubic aspiration and more than 100 cfu/ml from a catheter specimen is considered to be significant, but not if the patient has had a long-term catheter in situ, as these get colonized anyway. It is important to note that the absence of bacteriuria does not exclude an infection and the presence of vaginal epithelial cells suggests contamination.

Sterile pyuria

Pyuria has been defined as more than 10 wbc/mm^3 of urine and is generally indicative of an inflammatory response of the urothelium to bacterial invasion. Pyuria with a negative culture may suggest calculus disease, tuberculosis, tumour or incompletely or partially treated UTI or even ongoing antibiotic therapy. White cells can also be found in chlamydial urethritis, glomerulonephritis and interstitial cystitis. These conditions can elicit large numbers of fresh polymorphonuclear leucocytes in the urine and these are called glitter cells. In the presence of sterile pyuria, a repeat specimen should be sent and other investigations for the causes of the pyuria should be commenced. In the elderly, pyuria alone is not a good predictor of bacteriuria and pyuria is also not a significant finding post-instrumentation or post-catheterization of the urinary tract.

Treatment

Uncomplicated acute cystitis can be treated with urine culture and 3 days of antimicrobial therapy such as trimethoprim or a quinolone. It is important to take into account factors such as probable pathogens, recent hospitalization or instrumentation, side effects, patient allergy and cost. Cystitis complicated by any other factors should be treated with a 7–10 day course. It is also important to recognize any underlying factors that might suggest a complicated UTI. Groups at risk are the elderly, males, pregnant women, diabetics, immunocompromised people or those with an underlying functional or anatomic urinary tract anomaly.

The prevalence of bacteriuria is about 20% in those over 80 years of age. There is no indication to treat the elderly in the presence of bacteriuria that is asymptomatic.

In those with symptoms, the goal of treatment should be to eliminate the symptoms, as it may be impossible to eradicate the bacteriuria completely. The elderly should also be treated with a longer course of antibiotics: 7 days for those with cystitis and at least 14 days for those with pyelonephritis.

UTIs in men should be considered as complicated until proven otherwise. They may have underlying abnormalities such as prostatic hypertrophy, calculi, bladder tumour, urethral stricture, vesicoureteric reflux or pelviureteric junction obstruction. *E. coli* causes only 25% of infection in men as compared to 85% women. Treatment should consist of a course of antibiotics for 7–10 days, but if prostatitis is present, a 6-week course is recommended. In pregnant women, pyelonephritis is a risk factor for pre-term labour, therefore prompt diagnosis and aggressive treatment are warranted. Diabetics are at an increased risk of UTI compared to the normal population and they also have a higher risk of developing complications. Diabetics therefore require an aggressive approach to treatment, including intravenous antibiotics if there is any suggestion of pyelonephritis.

Pyelonephritis

Pyelonephritis is defined as inflammation of the renal parenchyma and pelvis. Patients usually present with fever with or without chills associated with loin pain and tenderness. Bacteraemia and sepsis are common; patients may also present with nausea, vomiting, diffuse abdominal pain and sometimes symptoms of cystitis. Routine blood tests along with cultures of blood and urine should be performed. *E. coli* causes 80% of pyelonephritis. An ultrasound of the renal tract is recommended in high-risk patients, especially if there is a suspicion of obstruction or if the patient is not responding to appropriate antimicrobial therapy. A CT scan may be more appropriate if further imaging is required. Oral antibiotics for 10–14 days is recommended, but if the patient is severely ill or has any underlying complicating factors, parenteral antibiotics are recommended. It is important to remember that there is a 10–30% relapse rate.

Emphysematous pyelonephritis is a severe necrotizing form of acute bacterial pyelonephritis in which gas is present, either within the kidney or in the perirenal space. The mortality rate is between 20–40% and diagnosis requires a high index of suspicion. In total, 70–90% of the cases occur in diabetics; it can also occur after a recent attack of pyelonephritis or in patients with obstructed kidneys. Patients may have a palpable flank mass and, rarely, surgical emphysema in the flank or thigh. *E. coli* is once again the causative organism but there can be other gas-forming organisms as well. Plain X-rays may demonstrate gas either in or around the kidney and CT scans are usually pathognomonic. Treatment is aimed at resuscitation, correction of diabetic status and antimicrobials. Nephrectomy is the treatment of choice after initial resuscitation; surgical removal reduces mortality rates to about 20%.

Fournier's gangrene

Fournier's gangrene is an acute urological emergency that should be recognized and treated immediately. It is a necrotizing infection involving the external genitalia, and perineum and can extend to the anterior abdominal wall. It carries a high mortality rate ranging between 50 and 80%. Patients are usually toxic and will have local evidence of infection. In addition, the important signs to note are crepitus and the presence of a black spot that might denote diffuse necrosis in the subcutaneous tissues.

Fournier's gangrene is usually seen in the immunocompromised and is caused by a synergistic infection comprising enteric Gram-negative organisms, Gram-positive staphylococci or streptococci and anaerobes. The infection results in obliterative endarteritis leading to widespread necrosis. Treatment includes resuscitative measures, antimicrobials and urgent surgical debridement that needs to be extensive. As the source of sepsis is usually urinary or colorectal, it is important to assess these systems and occasionally a suprapubic catheter or even a diverting colostomy may be required. A second-look debridement is recommended after 24 hours. Once the wound appears free of infection, skin grafting may be required.

Further reading

Common Infections and Infestations. Jefferson KP, MacDonaugh RP (eds). Mimms Handbook of Urology, 2nd edition. Haymarket Publications: London, 20045, Chapter 4, pp 53–66.

Smith J, Persad R, Smith P, Winder A. Keeping control: A practical guide to prevention and treatment of urinary incontinence. London: Vermillion, 2001: pp 66–9.

Trichomonas vaginalis

Arnold Fernandes

Introduction

Trichomoniasis is caused by *Trichomonas vaginalis* (TV); a flagellated protozoan. In women it is found in the vagina, urethra and paraurethral glands. In men, infection usually involves the urethra.

It is a common infection with an estimated 150–200 million cases globally each year. However, in the UK it is relatively uncommon with 6435 cases reported by English GUM clinics in 2003.

In adults, trichomoniasis is almost exclusively sexually transmitted, although there are anecdotal reports of transmission from fomites.

Presentation

Women

In women, TV can present with a vaginal discharge, vulval itchiness, dysuria or an offensive odour; however, 10–50% of women may be asymptomatic.

On examination there may be vulvitis or vaginitis. The vaginal discharge may vary in consistency from thin and scanty to thick and profuse. The pH of the discharge is usually > 4.5. The classically described frothy, yellow discharge occurs in only 10–30% of women.

The classic appearance of the 'strawberry cervix' on naked-eye examination often shown in text books is seen in only approximately 2% of infected women.

Some women will have no abnormalities on examination.

Men

Up to 50% of men with trichomoniasis are asymptomatic and they may present as sexual partners of infected women. In the symptomatic group of men, the presence of urethral discharge and/or dysuria is a common presentation. This may be indistinguishable from urethritis of other aetiologies.

Of infected men, 50–60% may present with a urethral discharge, which is usually small or moderate in amount. Rarely there may be associated balanoposthitis.

Often, in men presenting with symptoms of urethritis, TV cannot be detected (see below).

Complications

T. vaginalis infection is associated with pre-term delivery and low birth weight. TV is a cofactor for the transmission of HIV.

Diagnosis

Women

The gold standard test is culture, although this is no longer widely available. In primary care, send a high vaginal swab (HVS) to your lab. They will make a smear and stain it (e.g. with acridine orange or Leishman's stain). In GUM clinics the test used is wet-mount microscopy of a freshly obtained specimen. Many women are diagnosed with TV when the organism is discovered as an incidental finding when they are having cervical cytology. Stained microscopy has lower specificity than wet-mount microscopy; its positive predictive value is particularly low in low prevalence countries like the UK. If you get a TV diagnosis in a woman on a cytology report and she has had suggestive symptoms of the infection or multiple partners, then assume it is a true positive result. However, if for example she has been in a monogamous relationship for years, it is worthwhile confirming the diagnosis either by use of a HVS specimen and a different stain or referral to GUM for wet-mount microscopy.

PCR tests have been developed although they are not widely used yet. Point of care agglutination tests have also been developed and appear to perform well but will probably mostly be used in resource-poor countries.

Men

Diagnosis in men is hampered by the poor sensitivity of stained or wet-mount microscopy tests. Most male contacts are simply treated epidemiologically rather than being given a diagnosis.

Some men have their occult TV treated when their non-specific urethritis fails to improve with azithromycin and they are given metronidazole as a second-line agent (see NSU, page 146).

Even if available, urethral culture also has low sensitivity. When PCR tests are more widely available the situation might improve.

Treatment

A significant proportion of people infected with TV (thought to be 20–25%) may spontaneously clear the infection, however, of course, you cannot know if your patient is in this group and there is the potential for unpleasant symptoms and complications if left untreated. Because organisms can inhabit the female urethra, vaginal treatment alone cannot be relied upon.

Treatment options include:

- metronidazole 400 mg b.d. for 5 days
- metronidazole 2 g once
- tinidazole 2 g once.

The single dose has the advantage of improved compliance; however, there is some evidence to suggest that the failure rate is higher, especially if partners are not treated concurrently.

Patients treated with metronidazole should be advised not to take alcohol for the duration of treatment and for at least 48 hours afterwards because of the possibility of a disulfiram-like (Antabuse effect) reaction.

There is currently no effective alternative to imidazole compounds. The opinion of a specialist should be sought for patients who are known to have an allergy to these compounds. In cases of true allergy, desensitization should be considered.

Recurrent TV

In cases of treatment failure, it is important to check that the individual has been compliant to the treatment. Check also that the partner has been treated and exclude the possibility of re-infection. Patients who fail to respond to a first course of treatment often respond to a repeat course of standard treatment. Imidazole resistance is rare but will explain some treatment failures. Your lab might be able to do a resistance test. A double dose of metronidazole will often still work in this situation.

Treatment of sexual partners

Sexual partner(s) should be treated simultaneously, and sexual abstinence advised until treatment is completed. The opportunity should be taken to screen current sexual partners for other STIs.

See page 7 for advice on partner notification.

Pregnancy and breast feeding

While the safety of metronidazole in pregnancy is not established, the published data suggest no association with increased teratogenic risk.

Metronidazole can be used in all stages of pregnancy and during breast feeding. However, it is prudent to avoid metronidazole in the first trimester and high dose regimens are best avoided in pregnancy and during breast feeding. Metronidazole may make breast milk bitter.

For symptomatic relief in early pregnancy, local therapies (clotrimazole pessaries 100 mg daily for 7 days or Aci-jel) could be used, but systemic treatment will ultimately be necessary to eradicate the infection.

Neonatal infection of girls can occur but usually spontaneously resolve without treatment after several days because the organism is dependent on maternal oestrogens.

Sexual contacts

Screening for coexistent STIs should be undertaken in the index case and their sexual partners.

Sexual contacts should be treated epidemiologically (i.e. without waiting to see if you get a positive result) with the standard regimens above in order to limit the spread of infections.

Further reading

Sherrard J. UK 2001 national guideline on the management of *Trichomonas vaginalis* infection. http://www.bashh.org/guidelines/ceguidelines.htm

Vulvovaginal candidiasis

Arnold Fernandes

Introduction

Thrush is the common name used when *Candida* species cause vulvovaginal symptoms. Asymptomatic carriage should be referred to as candidosis. Vulvovaginal candidiasis is usually (80–90%) caused by *Candida albicans*. In a small minority of cases, non-albicans species such as *Candida glabrata* may be incriminated. The clinical features of the albicans and non-albicans species are however indistinguishable.

Presentation

Vulvovaginal candidiasis may be associated with vulval itchiness or vulval soreness. Some women may have a vaginal discharge that characteristically is described as being curdy and with at worst a mild smell.

The vulval soreness may contribute to superficial dyspareunia.

Examination of a woman with vulvovaginal candidiasis may reveal varying degrees of vulval erythema and oedema. The discharge may be seen in the vagina or coating the vaginal walls. In extreme cases, fissuring of the vulva may be seen. None of these symptoms or signs is specific for the diagnosis of candidiasis.

Candidiasis is often diagnosed on the basis of clinical features alone and as many as half of these women may have other conditions, e.g. allergic reactions. During their reproductive years, 10–20% of women may harbour *Candida* species in the absence of symptoms. These women do not require treatment.

Complications

There are no significant complications.

Diagnosis

Clinical

In most cases of women presenting in general practice settings, a diagnosis of candidiasis is made on clinical grounds.

The pH of vaginal fluid tends to remain acidic (4.0–4.5) in cases of candidiasis. (If pH > 4.5, suspect bacterial vaginosis/trichomoniasis).

Microscopic diagnosis

The diagnosis of candidiasis is confirmed by microscopy of a Gram-stained smear of discharge collected from anterior fornix or lateral vaginal wall. The presence of spores or pseudohyphae helps in confirming the diagnosis, although the sensitivity of microscopy is less than 65%.

Culture

Confirmation of the diagnosis by culture needs culture on Sabouraud's media. This should be considered in all symptomatic cases for which microscopy is inconclusive or identification of the species would be helpful, e.g. multiple previous treatments or concerns regarding the species involved. Since *Candida* species can be commensal organisms and grow easily, a positive culture does not mean that a woman's symptoms are due to the yeast.

Treatment

Treat only if symptomatic or if asymptomatic infection is present and antibiotics are being given for another indication.

A variety of preparations are available for the treatment of thrush. One simple and effective method (80–95% cure) is to give azole vaginal pessaries, e.g. clotrimazole 500 mg vaginal pessary as a single dose. If there is significant vulvitis, this can be combined with 1% clotrimazole cream applied to the vulva two or three times daily for up to 5–7 days, to relieve the vulval itch.

Clotrimazole cream on its own is of limited use.

Clotrimazole cream and pessaries can damage condoms, so alternative contraception should be used.

Alternatives to topical treatment are oral azoles, e.g. fluconazole as a single 150-mg oral dose or itraconazole (200 mg) taken twice a day for 1 day. These are no more effective than topical treatments. Oral therapies should be avoided in pregnancy or if there is any risk of an early pregnancy or if the woman is breast feeding.

Recurrent candidiasis

This is defined as four or more episodes of symptomatic candidosis annually. Prevalence is less than 5% of healthy women in their reproductive years. Pathogenesis of this condition is poorly understood. It is important to confirm that candidosis is really the cause of the symptoms – it could be another cause of chronic itch (see Genital itch, page 33)

Sometimes recurrent candidiasis is due to drug-resistant strains of *C. albicans* or to innately resistant species such as *C. glabrata* or *C. parapsilosis*. In recurring cases it is therefore important to ask your lab to determine the species and its antifungal sensitivity (fluconazole is the one usually tested against).

Regimens used are not based on randomized controlled trials. The basis of these regimens is induction with an anti-fungal agent, followed by a maintenance regimen for 4–6 months. Induction may involve using 200-mg clotrimazole pessaries for 3 days along with simultaneous topical use of clotrimazole cream, which is continued for 2 weeks or so. This is followed with the use of weekly clotrimazole 500-mg pessaries for 4–6 months or alternatively itraconazole 400 mg monthly for 4–6 months. Women on long-term oral antifungals should have their liver enzymes checked after a month.

Failure of routine antifungals to relieve symptoms can prove frustrating for both the patient and her practitioner. Referral to a specialist may sometimes be useful in these situations.

Candidiasis in pregnancy

Symptomatic candidiasis is more common in pregnant women than in non-pregnant women. Treatment with topical azoles is recommended and longer courses may be necessary. Oral therapy is contraindicated.

Sexual partner(s)

There is no evidence to support treatment of asymptomatic male partners.

Other management

General advice such as avoiding local irritants (perfumed soaps, deodorants, shower gel etc.) and avoiding tight-fitting synthetic clothing may prove helpful.

Warts

Steve Baguley

Introduction

Anogenital warts are very common – about 75 000 diagnoses were made by UK genitourinary medicine clinics in 2002. An unknown number of additional cases were diagnosed in primary care.

Almost all anogenital warts are caused by types 6 and 11 of the human papilloma virus (HPV). These types are different from those that cause genital cancers (includes types 16, 18, 31 and many more). They are also different from the types that cause warts on the hands (usually type 1), although there are occasional reports of apparent transmission of type 1 HPV from the hand to genital skin leading to the growth of warts. This is more likely if the person is immunosuppressed or a child. In one study, 2% of genital warts in adults were caused by HPV type 1–4 compared to 15% in children. Because HPV types 6 and 11 are site specific due to a preference for some feature of the genital epithelium, they are transmitted directly from one person's genitals to another's. Penetrative sex is not necessary and condoms offer only modest protection against transmission.

Having your anogenital skin infected with HPV is extremely common – it is estimated that over half the UK population will have a genital HPV infection at some point in their life. Not all those infections will be with types 6 or 11 and only about a fifth of those infected with one of those types will develop warts.

For such a common condition, surprisingly little is known about the natural history of non-oncogenic types of HPV. Following infection, HPV 6 and 11 DNA remains detectable in the skin for a mean of about 8 months, but it is unclear whether the virus is then completely cleared from the skin or whether it persists in some latent form, perhaps to be reactivated at a later date. It is possible that both situations can occur. It is also unclear why only some people develop warts following infection.

Presentation

Warts can occur at any site, although the posterior fourchette, perifrenular and perianal regions are the most likely places. This is because the virus finds easier entry to the skin in areas most likely to suffer minor trauma during sex and defecation. On thin, moist epithelium such as the urethral meatus, under the foreskin and the vagina/introitus, warts tend to be soft and non-keratinized. In other areas such as the perianal region or the shaft of the penis the warts can be quite keratinized. This has implications for treatment. Perianal warts are not an indication of receptive anal sex, although anal canal warts are.

Warts are usually skin coloured but can be redder on soft skin because the capillary loops within the wart show through. Occasionally, warts can be darker than the surrounding skin and so they can sometimes be confused with basal cell papillomata (aka sebaceous warts).

Sometimes, in hard-to-see areas such as the perianal area or within the urethra, warts are diagnosed because of symptoms other than their appearance. Perianal or anal warts can be very itchy or cause bleeding on defecation; urethral warts can cause haematuria. Occasionally vaginal or cervical warts are found when someone with low grade cervical intraepithelial neoplasia (CIN) attends for colposcopy.

Complications

Despite being so common, warts cause very few major problems. Very rarely they can grow so large as to obstruct the urethra, anus or vagina, thus making urination, defecation or childbirth difficult. The most common 'complication' is probably psychological distress leading to long-term sexual isolation. Even after the warts have gone, some people become fixated with the idea that they are redeveloping the lesions and require repeated reassurance and sometimes psychological input.

Children born to women with cervicovaginal HPV can sometimes develop laryngeal papillomatosis or genital warts. Although 'benign', laryngeal papillomas can occasionally cause laryngeal obstruction. It is therefore sensible to have as little wart tissue present at delivery as possible, although there is no evidence that doing so reduces the risk of neonatal complications.

The presence of vaginal warts does not increase a woman's chance of having high-grade CIN or cervical cancer. However, there is emerging evidence that perianal and anal warts might be associated with high-grade anal squamous intra-epithelial neoplasia. The significance and implications of this are unclear at present.

Diagnosis

Warts are usually diagnosed on the basis of their appearance – a lump with a roughened surface growing on the skin. The wart could be flat or protruding. Sometimes they can take on an atypical appearance or a normal feature of the skin could be mistaken for warts. If in doubt, the patient should be referred to someone with experience in diagnosing warts. This usually means a visit to the local GUM clinic. Rarely, a biopsy is needed to confirm the diagnosis.

Treatment

Although numerous treatments are available for warts, none are particularly effective, with cure rates in the region of 70–80%. Even when they disappear, there is about a 20% recurrence rate in the following 3 months. If the patient is immunosuppressed due to drugs, disease or pregnancy, clearance and recurrence rates are even worse.

Warts eventually clear spontaneously in most people, although the time to clearance varies from weeks to years. Therefore, it is usually worthwhile treating, although in awkward-to-get-at areas such as the anus or vagina there is an argument for leaving them alone if the person is happy with that and there is no risk of onward transmission.

Some treatment methods require repeated visits to the surgery/clinic and are therefore to be avoided. Here, a strategy is presented for maximizing success in wart eradication whilst avoiding numerous consultations and unnecessary cost.

A few warts anywhere

First-line treatment consists of freezing with liquid nitrogen or equivalent. Apply for 20 seconds and repeat three times. Try to create a halo of frozen skin around each wart. It is the thawing and refreezing that has the most effect.

Second-line treatment depends on the site – see below.

Many soft warts

For example, those located under the foreskin or the vaginal introitus. First-line treatment is podophyllotoxin 0.15% cream (trade name Warticon®). Apply twice daily for 3 days, then have a 4-day break before resuming if warts persist. Use for a maximum of 5 weeks before review.

Second-line treatment is imiquimod cream (Aldara®). Apply half or a whole sachet on alternate nights. Use for a maximum of 16 weeks with a review every 4–6 weeks.

Many keratinized warts

Many keratinized warts in an accessible site, e.g. the penile shaft, should be treated as follows.

First-line treatment is podophyllotoxin 0.5% liquid (Warticon® or Condyline®). Apply twice daily for 3 days, then have a 4-day break before resuming if warts persist. Use for a maximum of 5 weeks before review.

Second-line treatment is imiquimod cream (Aldara®). Apply half or a whole sachet on alternate nights. Use for a maximum of 16 weeks with review every 4–6 weeks. People often have to stop and start the treatment if it becomes too uncomfortable.

Urethral meatus

It is unusual for warts to extend more than about 1.5 cm into the urethra. Even so they can be tricky to treat. A narrow auroscope piece can be useful for seeing the extent of the lesions and if they extend to the limits of visibility, it is best to refer the person to a urologist for urethroscopy and treatment. More distal lesions can usually be treated in the clinic/surgery. A nasal speculum can be useful for this.

For first-line treatment, try careful freezing or podophyllotoxin 0.15% cream, as above.

For second-line treatment use electrocautery – bipolar diathermy is probably best.

Perianal warts

First-line treatment is imiquimod.

Second-line treatment is electrocautery, weekly freezing or surgery.

Cervical warts

It can be hard to confidently diagnose warty lesions on the cervix without a colposcope. It is therefore best to refer to your local colposcopy department for further investigation and perhaps biopsy.

- Patients should be warned that most treatments cause discomfort and local skin reactions.
- Podophyllotoxin is a cytotoxic agent derived from the root of the plant *Podophyllum peltatum*; it should definitely not be used during pregnancy.
- Imiquimod is a Toll receptor 7 ligand that induces an antiviral cytokine response in the skin. Its safety in pregnancy is unconfirmed.
- Freezing causes epidermal necrosis and is safe during pregnancy.
- If you choose to use a home treatment, make sure the patient knows which lumps are warts and which ones are just part of their normal skin.

Sexual contacts

There is no need to trace sexual contacts. People do not need to use condoms with current long-term partners since their partner will already have been exposed to the virus. People should be advised to avoid sex with new contacts until 3 months after the warts have gone. Condoms offer little protection against HPV acquisition.

Other management

Some people will have other STIs so they should be offered an STI screen.

If the patient shaves their genitals they should be advised to stop temporarily since the shaving nicks can give the virus easier access to the skin and encourage further wart growth.

Further reading

Maw R. UK national guideline for the management of anogenital warts. http://www.bashh.org/guidelines/hpv%2003%2002b.pdf

Index

pelvic inflammatory disease (PID)
(*cont.*)
  gonorrhoea 116
  management 156
  pregnancy 155
  presentation 153–4
  treatment 155
penile intra-epithelial neoplasia (PIN)
    113
permethrin 150, 163
phosphodiesterase (PDE-5) inhibitors
    101
Phthirus pubis 149–51
PID *see* pelvic inflammatory disease
PIN *see* penile intra-epithelial neoplasia
polycystic ovary syndrome (PCOS),
    infertility 139
POP *see* progesterone-only pill
pregnancy
  BV 89
  candidiasis, vulvovaginal 186
  Chlamydia trachomatis 95
  HIV/AIDS 135
  PID 155
  syphilis 174
  Trichomonas vaginalis (TV) 183
pregnancy, unwanted 66–73
priapism 157–8
progesterone-only pill (POP),
    contraception 20, 22, 26–7
prostatitis 159–61
psoriasis 34, 106
psychological causes, genital itch 34
pubic lice 34, 149–51
pyelonephritis 179
pyuria 178

rape 54–8
Reiter's syndrome 165–8
renal impairment, genital itch 34

SARA *see* sexually acquired reactive
    arthritis
SARCs *see* sexual assault referral
    centres
scabies 162–4
  genital itch 33

genital skin lumps 37
scrotal pain, differential diagnosis
    175–6
scrotal swellings 51–3
  epididymal cyst 51–2
  hydrocoele 51
  testicular cancer 52–3
  varicocoele 52
sebaceous glands, genital skin lumps
    37
sebaceous wart 38
sexual abuse 7–9
sexual assault 54–8
  consequences 56–7
  definitions 54–5
  incidence 55
  management 57–8
  perpetrator 55–6
  risk factors 55
sexual assault referral centres (SARCs)
    58
sexually acquired reactive arthritis
    (SARA) 165–8
spectinomycin 118
sterile pyuria 178
sterilization, contraception 24–5, 28
stress incontinence 48–50
surgical therapy, transgender patients
    62–3
syphilis 169–74
  complications 171
  diagnosis 171–3
  genital skin lumps 38
  management 174
  pregnancy 174
  presentation 169–71
  treatment 173

teenagers, contraception 17–20
testicular cancer 52–3
testicular torsion 175–6
thrush 34–5, 184–6
tinea cruris 35, 105–6
tinidazole 182
torsion, testicular 175–6
transgender patients 59–65
  diagnosis 60